The Primary Management
of Hand Injuries

THE PRIMARY MANAGEMENT OF HAND INJURIES

Campbell Semple FRCS
Consultant Hand Surgeon
Western Infirmary, Glasgow

Illustrated by **Martin Bone** BSc
Heriot Watt University, Edinburgh

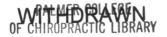
A Pitman Medical Publication
Distributed by

YEAR BOOK MEDICAL PUBLISHERS INC.
35 East Wacker Drive, Chicago

First published 1979

© Pitman Medical Publishing Co Ltd, 1979

This book is copyrighted in England and
may not be reproduced by any means
in whole or in part. Application with
regard to reproduction should be directed
to the copyright owner.

ISBN: 0—8151—7592—2

Library of Congress Cataloging in Publication Data

Semple, Campbell.
    The primary management of hand injuries.

    Bibliography: p.
    Includes index.
    1.   Hand—Wounds and injuries.   I.   Title.
[DNLM: 1.   Hand injuries—Therapy.   WE830 S473p]
RD559.S45   617.1   79—14127
ISBN 0—8151—7592—2

Code: WOH

Distributed in Continental North, South and
Central America, Hawaii, Puerto Rico and
The Philippines by
YEAR BOOK MEDICAL PUBLISHERS INC.
35 East Wacker Drive, Chicago, Illinois 60601
by arrangement with
Pitman Medical Publishing Co Ltd
PO Box 7, Tunbridge Wells,
Kent, TN1 1XH, England

Printed and bound in Great Britain
at The Pitman Press, Bath

INTRODUCTION

A large number of casual attenders at hospital emergency departments complain of injury to their hand. The majority of young
casualty officers have received little or no training in diagnosing or
treating these common problems; a considerable number of
significant injuries to the hand are missed in the casualty department; and injuries which are noted are often treated inappropriately,
with considerable inconvenience and upset to the patient.

This book is designed to cover these difficulties and to make
casualty officers aware of the problems, some minor some major,
passing through their hands daily, and to give them some basis of
knowledge and confidence to treat the patients more effectively.

It is hoped that this small book will function as a *vademecum*
rather than a textbook—carry it around with you, as you work,
and within a week or two you will have absorbed most of its
message and your patients will, hopefully, be benefiting.

In striving to keep this book brief and relevant, the hand
has been considered as beginning, or ending, at the wrist, and to
avoid becoming a textbook on tendon repairs, major skin loss and
the like, the conditions covered here are those capable of good
treatment in an emergency room or casualty department. When a
flexor tendon has been divided, this requires full operating facilities
and an experienced surgeon's skills; this level of injury and its
treatment is beyond the scope of this volume and although the
diagnosis is very much part of the casualty officer's work, the
formal treatment of these injuries should be referred to skilled
hand surgeons. The level at which problems are deemed important
enough to be referred onwards for further treatment will vary
from hospital to hospital, and the attitudes reflected in this book
are those of the Hand Surgery Unit based at the Western Infirmary,
Glasgow.

CONTENTS

Chapter 1

FRACTURES AND JOINT INJURIES

Most of the bones of the hand have a simple structure with a shaft containing medulla and two ends covered with articular cartilage; these bones have an excellent blood supply, and fractures of the fingers or metacarpal bones usually heal quickly and easily. A different situation exists in the carpus, however, where there are a number of small, more or less round bones which are largely covered by cartilage and have a rather precarious blood supply, and non-union or ischaemic necrosis of these bones does occur.

Direct injury to the hand, such as striking the fist against a wall, or a heavy weight falling on to the finger, produces either bruising of the soft tissues, or a fractured bone. A direct blow to the hand tends to produce either a transverse fracture of the neck or shaft of a phalanx or metacarpal, whereas a crushing injury results in a splintered or comminuted fracture. Indirect force applied to the hand such as a severe twisting injury to a finger is liable to produce a spiral or oblique fracture, or damage to the soft tissues in and around a finger joint.

These various types of injury produce characteristic displacements of the fracture fragments, due more to the varying pulls of the surrounding anatomical structures than to the original trauma force. For example the common fracture of the *neck* of the 5th metacarpal always results in a flexion deformity of the distal fragment, the head of the 5th metacarpal, due to the pull of the hypothenar muscles and the flexor tendon. A fracture of a metacarpal *shaft* tends not to displace to any serious degree, as it is splinted in position by the neighbouring normal metacarpal. Fractures of the proximal phalanx are very prone to displace, and can be extremely difficult to reduce and hold; these injuries are dealt with more fully on page 20. The spiral, or oblique, fracture which follows a severe twisting strain to a finger is liable to result in shortening and malrotation of the finger, as the two fracture fragments slide on each other under the pull of the long flexor and extensor tendons. This tendency of spiral fractures to produce rotatory deformities must be watched for, as the finger may end up with an awkward tendency to cross over a neighbouring finger on flexion, if not fully reduced initially.

Injuries of the carpal bones are caused by a fall on the outstretched hand, or a blow to the base of the thumb. These fractures are often difficult to detect radiologically, but can lead to considerable damage to the wrist joint region if inadequately treated; these injuries are dealt with more fully on page 16.

Indirect trauma to a finger is very prone to produce a dislocation or other injury to a joint, either the metacarpophalangeal, or the proximal interphalangeal joint. It is important to appreciate the basic anatomy of these joints in order to understand and interpret clinical and X-ray changes in the fingers.

8

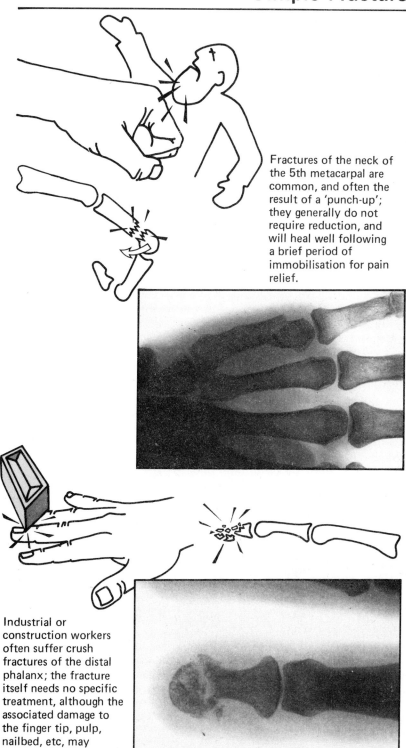

Fractures of the neck of the 5th metacarpal are common, and often the result of a 'punch-up'; they generally do not require reduction, and will heal well following a brief period of immobilisation for pain relief.

Industrial or construction workers often suffer crush fractures of the distal phalanx; the fracture itself needs no specific treatment, although the associated damage to the finger tip, pulp, nailbed, etc, may require repair.

All finger joints consist essentially of two cartilage covered bone ends held together by a joint capsule; this capsule is strengthened however on both sides and on the volar surface. The collateral ligaments of finger joints will be damaged by undue lateral stress on the joint, and the volar plate, a condensation of fibro-cartilage on the palmar aspect of the joint capsule, will be damaged by excessive hyperextension of the joint.

Moderate traumatic deformation of a finger joint will produce a 'sprained' joint; this means that the ligaments have been stretched but not ruptured, and there is usually some bleeding into the joint cavity and bruising round it. With a more severe strain on the joint, a collateral ligament may rupture, or the volar plate may tear. These ruptures of capsular structures produce marked swelling and pain around the joint, together with instability. It may not be possible to demonstrate the joint instability without first anaesthetising the finger and then taking X-ray films with the joint stressed to show the excessive ligament laxity. When a volar plate or collateral ligament tears, it generally does so at one end, and there is often a tiny, but significant, fragment of bone to be seen at the margin of the joint on a plain X-ray film. Do not ignore these small fragments. They are not 'small chip or flake fractures' . . . they imply that the joint has been badly damaged and requires careful management if it is to regain normal function.

Similarly, when dealing with a dislocated finger joint, it must be appreciated that these ligaments will have been badly stretched, if not actually ruptured by the dislocation, and will require to be treated after the dislocation is reduced. If a dislocated finger reduces with an obvious snap, the joint ligaments are probably intact, but if the joint reduces slackly and tends to displace again, then ligaments are probably damaged. However, if a dislocated joint is difficult or impossible to reduce, it generally means that the head of the proximal bone has 'button-holed' through part of the capsule or volar plate of the joint. If a joint cannot be reduced by close manipulation under good local anaesthesia, then further attempts should not be made, and surgical advice should be sought regarding the advisability of an open reduction of the joint.

With a sprained joint, or other injury where the ligaments and volar plate are intact, treatment will consist of resting the joint in the position of function, as described at the end of the chapter, until the swelling and pain have settled, and then commencing active movements of the joint. Straightforward injuries of finger joints should settle over a week or two, but if there appears to be undue stiffness or pain, an orthopaedic opinion should be sought. All patients with evidence of ligament/volar plate damage, such as small juxta-articular bone fragments, or undue joint laxity, should be seen by an orthopaedic or hand surgeon, as there is often a case for operative repair of the damaged ligament. The ulnar collateral ligament of the thumb is particularly prone to this type of tear, following a fall on the outstretched thumb; an awkward fall on a trampoline, or while ski-ing often produces such a ligament tear.

Finger Joint Injuries

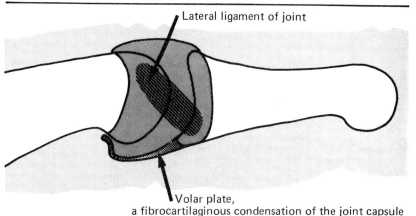

Lateral ligament of joint

Volar plate,
a fibrocartilaginous condensation of the joint capsule

A sprained joint is
swollen and painful due
to contained blood.

Soft tissue swelling and
blood in the dislocated
joint

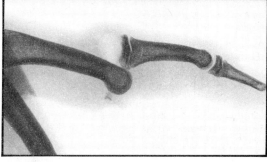

Volar plate avulsion
fracture.

Abduction strain of the
metacarpophalangeal
joint of the thumb may
tear the ulnar collateral
ligament, with a small
avulsion fracture from
the base of the proximal
phalanx.

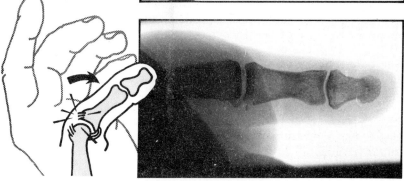

It is not easy to separate fractures of the hand into those which require specialist treatment and those which can be easily dealt with in the casualty department; the following categories are suggested as guidelines however.

The 'zone of problem fractures' runs from the heads of the metacarpals to the base of the middle phalanx. Any fracture occurring in this zone is likely to give rise to further problems and further advice should be sought. This zone also includes the entire base of the thumb from the trapezium out to the base of the proximal phalanx.

It must be stressed that *any* fractures in this area, no matter how small or apparently insignificant, are likely to give rise to some difficulty in management, and elsewhere in this chapter the specific problems of joint fractures (proximal phalanx and carpal injuries) are described.

Another way of looking at this problem zone is to consider it as encompassing the metacarpophalangeal and proximal interphalangeal joints; fracture damage in this area is therefore likely to interfere with the normal movement of these joints and compromise the long term function of the hand. Once a metacarpophalangeal joint or proximal interphalangeal joint has become stiff as a result of previous bone or soft tissue injury it can be extremely difficult, and often impossible, to correct. Hence the stress which we place on the diagnosis and treatment of fractures and joint damage in this area.

Fractures outside this zone, that is in the distal half of the fingers and in the region of the shafts of the metacarpals and most of the carpus, rarely give rise to much trouble and can usually be dealt with satisfactorily by simple splintage in the casualty department. If in doubt, however, an orthopaedic opinion should be sought. These rules apply to single fractures only and where multiple fractures of the hand exist, considerable force will have occurred, such as a heavy crushing injury, and specialist orthopaedic advice is necessary.

Other than in the problem zone, single fractures of the metacarpal shafts, for example, are rarely displaced, and will usually heal up easily within a week or two. Fractures at the end of the finger in the region of the distal interphalangeal joint or the phalanx, rarely give rise to much trouble, although the patient may have a rather stiff distal interphalangeal joint.

Fractures in the non-problem zone should therefore be treated on the basis of the patient's symptoms; if the hand is particularly painful or swollen, then good comfortable well-positioned splinting will be necessary, whereas some fractures of the metacarpal or terminal phalanx produce minimal symptoms and require little treatment beyond reassurance.

When assessing injuries to the carpus it should be appreciated that the common fractures or dislocations occur on the radial aspect, and injuries to the ulnar carpal bones, that is the pisiform, triquetral, hamate and capitate, are all rare. The specific problems of some of the carpal bones and the proximal phalanx are dealt with on the following pages.

Hand Fractures: Problem Zones

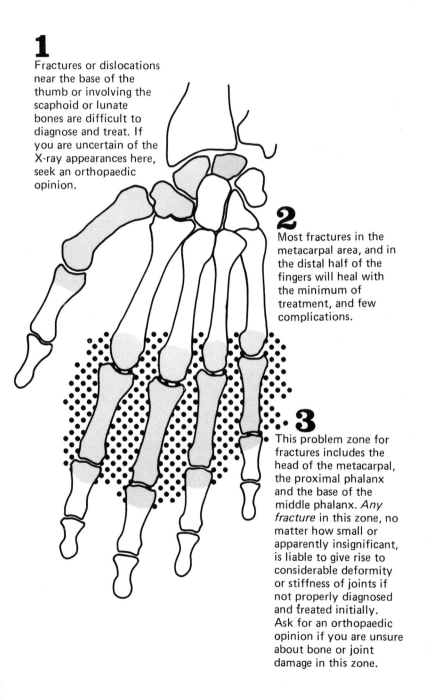

1
Fractures or dislocations near the base of the thumb or involving the scaphoid or lunate bones are difficult to diagnose and treat. If you are uncertain of the X-ray appearances here, seek an orthopaedic opinion.

2
Most fractures in the metacarpal area, and in the distal half of the fingers will heal with the minimum of treatment, and few complications.

3
This problem zone for fractures includes the head of the metacarpal, the proximal phalanx and the base of the middle phalanx. *Any fracture* in this zone, no matter how small or apparently insignificant, is liable to give rise to considerable deformity or stiffness of joints if not properly diagnosed and treated initially. Ask for an orthopaedic opinion if you are unsure about bone or joint damage in this zone.

SCAPHOID FRACTURES

The scaphoid bone, on the radial aspect of the carpus, lies partly in the proximal row of carpal bones, and partly in the distal row. A fall on the outstretched hand, usually in fit young men, causes hyperextension of the radio-carpal joint, and the dorsal lip of the radius may break the waist of the scaphoid bone; the patient will then present with a painful and tender wrist, particularly in the 'anatomical snuff box', between the end of the radius and the base of the thumb. X-ray films of this area are not easy to interpret and you should always have three views of the wrist to look at, an AP, a lateral and an oblique view. In a displaced fracture of the scaphoid the injury is obvious, but often the fracture is undisplaced, and the fine fracture line may not be seen on the initial films. If you are uncertain about the scaphoid bone it is better to be cautious and treat the wrist in plaster, and review it with fresh X-rays in the fracture clinic a few weeks later. The fracture line may then be apparent, or a visible difference in density between the two poles of the scaphoid may be seen. The proximal pole of the scaphoid has a rather precarious blood supply, and if the fracture does not heal satisfactorily this fragment may collapse and lead to second-ary osteoarthritic changes in the wrist joint. Careful primary treatment of these injuries can usually prevent this complication occurring, but it requires the casualty officer to detect the fracture initially, and if he is uncertain about the clinical or X-ray appearance he should support the wrist and thumb in a plaster cast and seek an orthopaedic or hand surgical opinion.

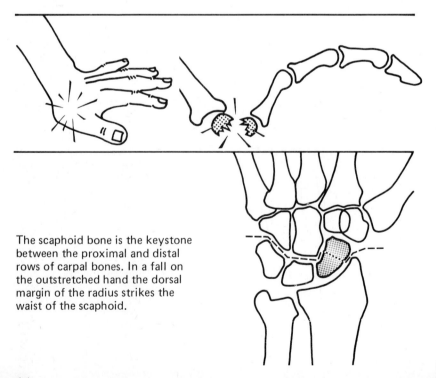

The scaphoid bone is the keystone between the proximal and distal rows of carpal bones. In a fall on the outstretched hand the dorsal margin of the radius strikes the waist of the scaphoid.

Carpal Scaphoid Fractures

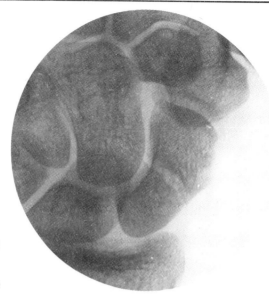

The X-ray above shows a fresh undisplaced fracture of the scaphoid with a fine line running across the waist of the bone. Such fractures are often difficult to see, and may be more apparent a few weeks later, as in the film on the right, when the relative ischaemia of the proximal pole shows up as a radio-dense fragment.

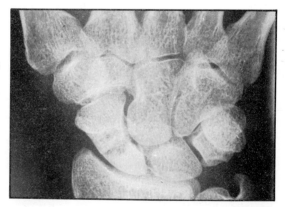

The lower film shows the late result of an untreated fracture of the scaphoid, with avascular collapse of the proximal pole, and marked osteoarthritic degeneration in the radio-scaphoid joint.

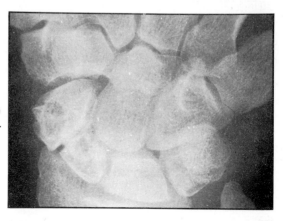

Bennett's Fracture

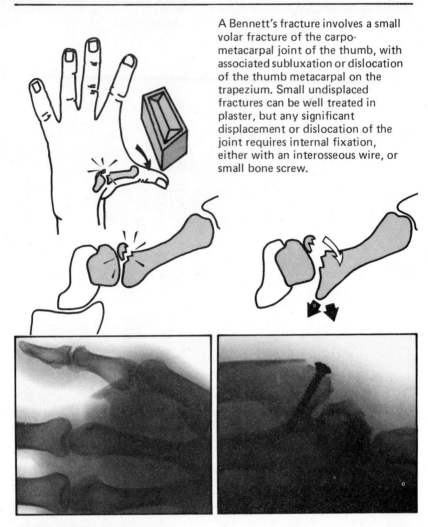

A Bennett's fracture involves a small volar fracture of the carpo-metacarpal joint of the thumb, with associated subluxation or dislocation of the thumb metacarpal on the trapezium. Small undisplaced fractures can be well treated in plaster, but any significant displacement or dislocation of the joint requires internal fixation, either with an interosseous wire, or small bone screw.

BENNETT'S FRACTURE

This is the name given to a fracture dislocation of the carpo-metacarpal joint of the thumb. It usually occurs in adults following an extension injury to the thumb, and is really a variety of volar plate injury, as described with joint injuries of the fingers. The small spur on the volar/flexor aspect of the base of the first meta-carpal is fractured, and the metacarpal and entire thumb then tends to dislocate proximally, under the considerable pull of the long flexor and extensor tendons of the thumb. This diagnosis should be suspected when there is pain, bruising, tenderness and often crepitus and instability at the base of the thumb. Proper treatment of this injury can be difficult, and may require operative fixation of the fracture, and an orthopaedic opinion should be sought.

On an AP view the
normal lunate is
surrounded by a clear
1 mm zone representing
articular cartilage; loss
of this regular
appearance should
suggest dislocation, and
will be confirmed on
careful study of a lateral
film of the wrist.

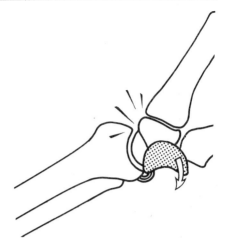

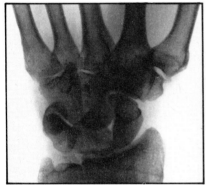

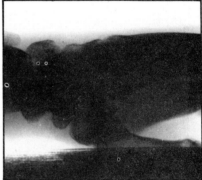

DISLOCATION OF THE CARPAL LUNATE

This injury is not common, but it is not easy to diagnose, as the
X-ray appearances are unusual. It occurs in young fit people
following a severe blow on the hyperextended wrist; this is a
somewhat similar mechanism to that causing a fracture of the
scaphoid, and occasionally both injuries may occur together, a
trans-scaphoid perilunate dislocation of the wrist. The lunate
bone generally dislocates anteriorly, and although no obvious
bump is present, the displaced bone may cause pressure symptoms
on the median nerve in the carpal tunnel. On an AP view of the
wrist, all the carpal bones have neat little lines, like canals, around
them, and the lunate bone should look like a wedge of cheese.
When the lunate is dislocated this regular appearance is altered on
the AP view, and a lateral view will confirm the anterior dislocation and rotation of the lunate bone. This injury generally
requires prompt surgical treatment to relieve the pressure on the
median nerve, and to minimise damage to the blood supply of the
lunate, and urgent orthopaedic advice should be sought.

THE METACARPAL REGION

Fractures of the shaft or neck of a metacarpal bone rarely give rise to much difficulty. These fractures often result from the use of the closed fist in a fight, and the patient may have few symptoms, apart from a rather bruised and swollen hand or knuckle. Spiral fractures of metacarpals are often difficult to see on an X-ray, and AP, lateral and oblique views of the hand should be requested to avoid missing these injuries. It is unusual for these fractures to require reduction, and comfortable splintage in the 'position of function' for a week or so will allow healing to commence, and then active movements can be encouraged.

It is tempting to try and reduce a fracture of the neck of the 5th metacarpal—a boxer's fracture—as they always lead to a flexion deformity at the fracture site. Achieving a closed reduction is difficult, and maintaining the reduction is virtually impossible, and attempts to hold a reduction in a plaster splint with pressure pads are very prone to produce a painful and stiff hand and little finger. If left to heal in the displaced position, the patient has an obvious bump of callus on the back of his hand, but this settles during the following 6 months or so, and function of the metacarpophalangeal joint of the little finger is rarely affected.

Occasionally, a transverse fracture of the metacarpal shaft, if badly displaced, may need reduction, and possibly internal fixation with a wire, but generally metacarpal shaft fractures are only slightly displaced and are stable, being splinted by the neighbouring normal metacarpal bones. With an oblique or spiral fracture of a metacarpal shaft, there is the risk that the metacarpophalangeal joint may unite with some slight rotation present, which might allow the fingers to cross when flexed; this complication can be avoided by making sure that the fingers are splinted in moderate flexion, as described at the end of this chapter.

These comments do not apply to the thumb metacarpal bone however, as it is an independent bone, unsupported by the other metacarpals. Any fracture of the first metacarpal, no matter how small, should be considered as a problem fracture, and referred for orthopaedic advice.

Metacarpal Fractures

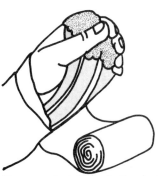

Firm comfortable splinting in the position of function will support and ease most fractures of the metacarpals.

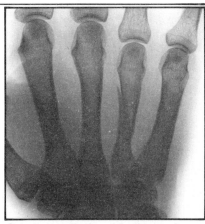

Spiral or undisplaced fractures of a metacarpal shaft can be difficult to see on an AP film.

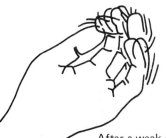

After a week or so, when the pain and swelling have settled, active mobilisation of the fingers should be encouraged.

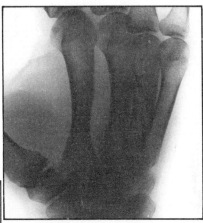

An oblique X-ray film will usually reveal metacarpal shaft fractures.

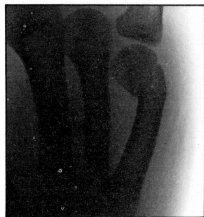

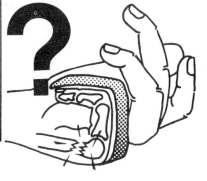

The common fracture of the neck of the 5th metacarpal produces a characteristic flexion deformity of the head of the bone, but attempts to reduce and hold these fractures generally produce increased pain and stiff hands.

THE PROXIMAL PHALANX

Single fractures of the proximal phalanx are generally either transverse or oblique.

If a transverse fracture is undisplaced, it may be possible to treat it by comfortable splintage in the position of function, but it is not sufficient to simply splint the one injured finger, and the neighbouring fingers should be included in the splintage. A careful watch should be kept on this fracture over the first week to 10 days to make quite certain that it is not displaced, and after 2 to 3 weeks the fracture should be well on the way to healing and gentle active movements may be started.

One of the difficulties in managing fractures of the proximal phalanx is that of obtaining good X-ray pictures; PA views are simple enough, but a true lateral view is often masked by the superimposed shadows of the other fingers. When dealing with finger fractures therefore, it is better to obtain oblique views in addition to the standard AP and lateral projections. If there is any significant dorsal angulation or displacement of the fracture fragment, then an orthopaedic or hand surgery opinion should be sought, as operative reduction and internal fixation of the fracture will probably be necessary.

A spiral or oblique fracture of the proximal phalanx, resulting from an excessive torque or strain on the finger, has a tendency to produce rotational deformity, so that the finger tips cross when the patient makes a fist. In a relatively undisplaced fracture it may be possible to control this tendency during the healing phase by taping neighbouring fingers in flexion, but if the fracture is at all displaced, open operation and internal fixation may be preferable. Do not forget to look for small fragments at the margins of joints, particularly metacarpophalangeal or proximal interphalangeal joints; these small fragments imply significant joint damage, usually involving a tear of a collateral ligament or volar plate, and will need careful supervision in the hand or fracture clinic, or operative repair if joint stiffness is to be avoided.

Fractures of the proximal interphalangeal joint itself, either involving the head of the proximal phalanx or the base of the middle phalanx, must be treated with extreme caution. Any articular fracture is very liable to lead to considerable joint stiffness and osteoarthritis, and the proximal interphalangeal joint is no exception. These small fractures can be extremely difficult to deal with, and generally result in some degree of joint stiffness, but with careful surgical management it may be possible to realign the joint surfaces and avoid serious stiffness of the joint.

In children, the epiphyseal region at the base of a phalanx may be injured, generally producing a mild angulation deformity at the fracture site. These deformities are extremely difficult to straighten out by closed manipulation, although one can occasionally manage it on the day of injury. One must remember, however, that these growth plates can adapt very rapidly to such a deformity, and the apparent deformity on X-ray generally grows out over the ensuing few months.

Proximal Phalanx Fractures

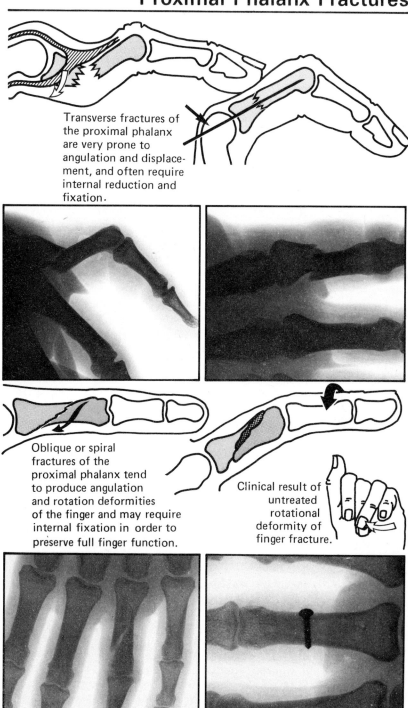

Transverse fractures of the proximal phalanx are very prone to angulation and displacement, and often require internal reduction and fixation.

Oblique or spiral fractures of the proximal phalanx tend to produce angulation and rotation deformities of the finger and may require internal fixation in order to preserve full finger function.

Clinical result of untreated rotational deformity of finger fracture.

PRINCIPLES OF TREATMENT

If the fracture or joint injury appears to be a problem one, as described before, then you should seek orthopaedic advice. The majority of fractures in the hand, however, are straightforward ones without undue displacement, and require simple splintage only until the pain has settled, after which active mobilisation should be encouraged. It is better to over-splint the hand initially, as the patient's complaint is generally of pain, and it is very much more comfortable to splint the whole hand rather than try to splint one finger only. Most fractures or sprains of the hand will become pain free within a few days, and mobilisation in a crepe bandage or other simple support can then be encouraged. Some patients, particularly elderly patients, may require the support of splintage for a longer time, but the same principles exist in that one should achieve a comfortable hand, and then start fingers moving actively.

It is important, however, that the hand should be splinted in a sensible fashion, so that when the patient starts moving the fingers again he can actually use the hand. It is a mistake to splint the fingers in an abnormal position; there is no place for splinting a finger either fully straight or fully flexed. If a fracture requires this kind of position in order to stabilise it, it would probably be better fixed internally by operation. Most simple fractures of the hand can be managed perfectly well with the hand as a whole being splinted in the position of function. This means that the wrist should be extended, the metacarpophalangeal and interphalangeal joints flexed, and the thumb brought across into opposition. If you study your own hand in its natural resting position, you will find that it lies in this position, and that the thumb tip tends to oppose to the index and middle finger. The hand which is splinted in this position should be comfortable, and this, together with elevation, should allow the swelling and inflammation around the fracture site to resolve rapidly; the patient should still be able to use the thumb and finger tips for minor activities. As the fracture heals and the pain and swelling resolve, an increase in movement will develop in the fingers, and in the case of most simple fractures in the hand, after a week of this splintage, the hand can be simply supported with a mild compressive bandage and increasing active movement can be encouraged.

From time to time one comes across a hand which becomes extremely stiff, swollen and painful, and may indeed proceed to a severe condition known as sympathetic dystrophy or Sudeck atrophy. Once this condition is established, it can be very difficult indeed to treat and many months of difficulty for the patient and for the physiotherapist are necessary; it is very much better to prevent this condition occurring by keeping a gentle eye on patients with an injured hand for the first couple of weeks to make sure that the pain and swelling of the fracture is settling comfortably and that the patient is beginning to use the hand. If there is any suggestion that this steady course of events is not occurring, then an orthopaedic opinion should be sought.

Principles of Treatment of Fractures

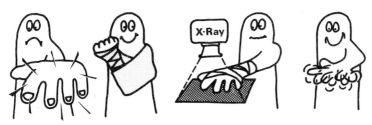

Straightforward fractures of the hand should have the symptoms relieved by comfortable splintage and elevation, and once the position of the fracture has been checked, by X-ray, splintage should remain for a week or so and active mobilisation of the hand and fingers commenced.

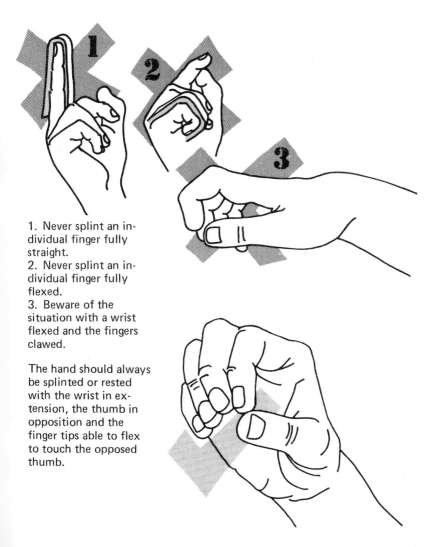

1. Never splint an individual finger fully straight.
2. Never splint an individual finger fully flexed.
3. Beware of the situation with a wrist flexed and the fingers clawed.

The hand should always be splinted or rested with the wrist in extension, the thumb in opposition and the finger tips able to flex to touch the opposed thumb.

REDUCTION AND SPLINTAGE

All dislocations in the hand should be reduced promptly, and if you cannot manage to reduce the dislocation after one attempt under good local anaesthesia, then refer the patient for further opinion. Further attempts at reducing a difficult dislocation will probably be prevented by a portion of ligament or tendon between the bone ends, and repeated attempts at reducing it may well produce further damage to the joint. With such interposition of soft tissues between bone ends, an open operation will be necessary to produce proper reduction of the dislocation. When a dislocation has been reduced, it should feel stable without any tendency to re-dislocate, but if you feel the joint is still unstable, then this should raise the question of a tear of a ligament or volar plate, and again further advice should be sought. If the joint feels stable, however, the affected finger, together with the neighbouring digits, should be rested comfortably in a splint in the position of function.

Similarly, with fractures in the hand, the aim should be to rest the injured finger or bone, together with its neighbouring digits, and possibly the whole hand, comfortably in the position of function. There are not many situations where reduction of a displaced fracture in an emergency room is advisable; if the displacement is slight, then reduction is probably not necessary, and if the displacement is significant, then reducing it and holding it by simple external splintage is generally difficult or impossible, and open operation may be necessary.

Various forms of splintage of the fingers and hand are available, but we prefer to use plaster of Paris splints, usually applied as a volar slab. Some hospitals like to use malleable splints made of aluminium, but we find that these tend to splint one finger only, and the edges of the aluminium often dig into the patient's hand in an uncomfortable manner. We find that a plaster of Paris splint laid on the volar aspect of a patient's hand gives a very comfortable bed for the injured fingers, including the digit on either side of the injured one. This sort of plaster applied for about a week usually produces a comfortable, pain free hand, which can then be adequately mobilised, often with the aid of a mild elastic, or crepe bandage.

As an intermediate stage in mobilising a finger, a small tubular bandage, or piece of tape, is used to attach an injured finger to a neighbouring normal finger which will allow gentle active mobilisation of the injured digits (buddy taping).

A support behind the wrist encourages the hand to adopt the position of function.

A volar plaster slab, approximately five to six layers thick, from the elbow to the fingertips is measured over a layer of gauze or plaster wool padding.

The wet plaster of Paris is laid on the volar aspect of the forearm and palm, and as it is drying one or two ridges are raised on it to provide maximum strength.

The plaster splint is comfortably bandaged in position as it dries using a crepe or mild elastic bandage.

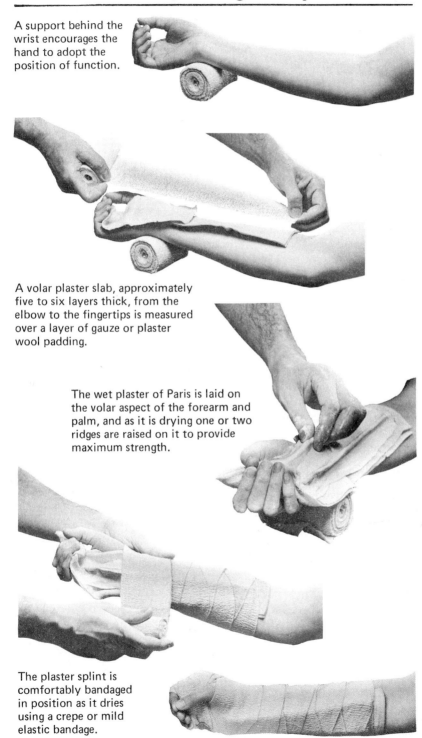

Chapter 2

THE CUT HAND:
TENDONS AND NERVES

The cut or bleeding hand is a very common problem, and if the skin alone is divided, then this type of wound is easily repaired in the casualty department, with full return of function in the hand. Once again, you must find out what caused the injury, as this will lead to suspicion of hidden problems in the wound and prevent a mis-diagnosis or bad treatment. For example, a transverse laceration on the palm of the hand which has been caused by a roller press machine is almost certainly a de-gloving injury and if not skilfully treated by an experienced surgeon will lead to the loss of a large portion of the palmar skin. A similar type of transverse palmar incision caused by a bread knife is very likely to have divided some significant tendons and nerves and this sort of wound again must be referred for expert advice. It is important to have a knowledge of some areas of anatomy in the hand, and to know how to examine the hand simply, without upsetting the patient or doing any further damage.

BLEEDING

All bleeding from the forearm or hand will stop given *moderate pressure on the wound and elevation.* There is *never* any case for exploring the wound in the emergency room and putting artery forceps or other instruments into it; this will almost certainly do further damage and alarm the patient and is quite unnecessary. If a proximal tourniquet has been applied to the arm, this should be removed, as this generally does more harm than good, and even if a significant artery, such as the radial artery, has been divided, this will not bleed to any significant degree if a clean dressing is applied to the wound and supported by moderate pressure from a crepe bandage, and the whole arm elevated for quarter of an hour.

It is important to reassure the patient at this stage, as most patients are naturally nervous and alarmed at the prospect of the bleeding from the hand, the pending sutures, and the pain which examination of the hand may cause. Once the bleeding has been controlled, it is only necessary to have a quick look *at* the wound, and not *in* it. There is nothing to be gained from poking around in a wound to see whether tendons or nerves have been divided. You should gain a quick look at the wound and note its extent, and where it lies anatomically, and then cover up the wound with a simple dressing, preferably one that can be removed easily, such as a tulle gras dressing or a moist Hibitane dressing. Once the wound has been neatly and comfortably covered, the hand can be examined distal to the wound; any damage to significant structures in the wound can be detected by distal examination. In the case of a sharp laceration on the front of the wrist, it may not be possible

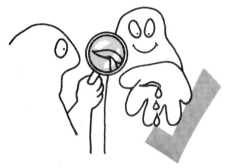

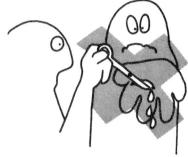

Always look *at* a wound and not *in* it.

You are always likely to do harm by poking around in a wound.

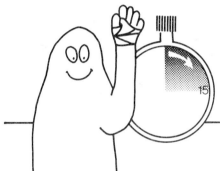

A bleeding wound should be controlled by a simple pressure dressing, elevation and time. There is no case for inserting haemostats or other instruments into a wound of the hand to control haemorrhage.

Once you have noted the anatomical situation of the wound and controlled the bleeding by means of a dressing, it is then possible to carefully and gently examine the hand distally and thereby assess the likely damaged structures in the wound. If any significant nerves or tendons have been divided in the wound, it should be possible to diagnose these by appropriate examination of the fingers.

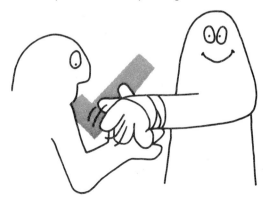

to make an exact list of all the structures divided, but it should certainly be possible to assess that the median nerve and a number of tendons have been divided, and the final diagnosis of the exact structures damaged can wait until the patient is fully anaesthetised in the operating theatre.

THE FRONT OF THE WRIST

This area is often cut when someone falls on their outstretched hand on a broken bottle, and self-inflicted wounds caused by would-be suicide attempts often damage structures in this area. All the important tendons and nerves to the hand pass through the front of the wrist, and if the cut is deep enough, then all of these structures can be divided. In general, if a person falls with most of their body weight behind them on to a sharp object such as a knife or broken glass, then a deep cut results involving tendons and nerves, whereas a glancing blow on the front of the wrist or a self-inflicted cut is generally much more superficial and may only damage the median nerve, lying just under the skin. Lacerations may of course occur in any depth and direction, but there is a tendency for most cuts to lie either on the anterior aspect of the wrist or on the ulnar aspect.

With lacerations on the anterior aspect of the wrist, the most superficial structure here is the palmaris longus tendon which is not itself important, but it must be appreciated that the median nerve lies immediately beneath it, and occasionally the palmaris longus tendon may be absent, in which case the median nerve is directly underneath the skin. Any wound therefore that goes deeper than the skin on the front of the wrist should be considered as a possible case of damage to the median nerve, and should be carefully assessed with this in mind. Deep to the median nerve lie the superficial flexor tendons to the fingers, and deep to them lie the profundus tendons. On the radial aspect of the median nerve lies the flexor carpi radialis tendon, and then just lateral to this lies the radial artery. If the cut is deep enough then all of these structures can be divided and will require very careful and painstaking repair by a surgeon experienced in hand surgery. With such deep lacerations there is no problem in diagnosing that a number of structures have been divided, but be on your guard to avoid missing a division or partial division of the median nerve, as often the most apparently superficial of lacerations on the front of the wrist has, in fact, damaged this structure.

THE ULNAR ASPECT OF THE WRIST

Lacerations in this region will initially damage the flexor carpi ulnaris tendon, and lying immediately deep to this tendon are the ulnar artery and ulnar nerve. The ulnar nerve, being protected by the strong flexor carpi ulnaris tendon, is less likely to be damaged by small superficial lacerations, but if there is any suggestion that the flexor carpi ulnaris tendon has been damaged, then one must also make sure that the underlying ulnar nerve has not been cut. A larger, or deeper, laceration on the ulnar aspect of the wrist may also involve some of the superficial and deep flexor tendons which lie to the radial side of the ulnar nerve.

The Front of the Wrist

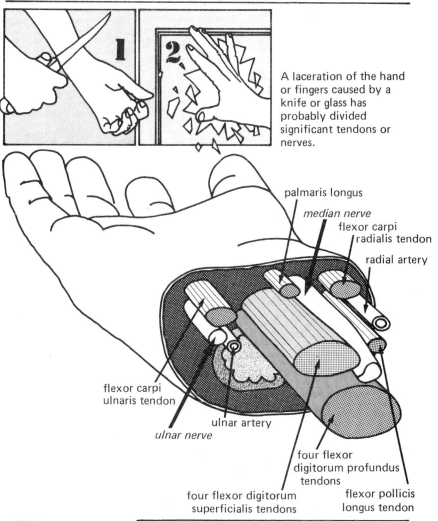

A laceration of the hand or fingers caused by a knife or glass has probably divided significant tendons or nerves.

palmaris longus

median nerve

flexor carpi radialis tendon

radial artery

flexor carpi ulnaris tendon

ulnar nerve

ulnar artery

flexor carpi ulnaris tendon

four flexor digitorum profundus tendons

four flexor digitorum superficialis tendons

flexor pollicis longus tendon

All these structures may be easily divided by a sharp wound on the front of the wrist. In particular it must be stressed how central and superficial is the median nerve, lying just under the skin and lying deep to, but not really protected by, the palmaris longus tendon.

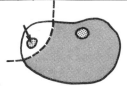

Deep wounds on the ulnar border of the wrist generally divide the flexor carpi ulnaris tendon, the ulnar nerve and artery and a varying number of the superficial and profundus tendons to the fingers.

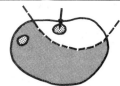

Lacerations on the anterior aspect of the wrist generally divide the median nerve, flexor carpi radialis tendon and a varying number of superficial and profundus tendons to the fingers.

THE BACK OF THE WRIST

Twelve tendons cross the dorsum of the wrist and they are all liable to be divided through lacerations in this region; the only other structure of note is the terminal branch of the radial nerve. Loss of sensation following division of the nerve is not important— often it is a square centimetre or so at the base of the thumb–it is more important, however, to be aware of these small nerve branches when carrying out surgery on the dorso-radial aspect of the wrist, as inadvertent division, crushing or ligature of the nerve may lead to troublesome and painful neuromata.

There are three groups of tendons in the twelve extensors of the wrist. Extensor carpi ulnaris, extensor carpi radialis longus and extensor carpi radialis brevis; the three extensors of the thumb, abductor pollicis longus, extensor pollicis brevis and extensor pollicis longus; and the extensors of the fingers, extensor digitorum communis (four tendons), extensor digiti minimi, extensor indicis proprius.

The most commonly divided tendons are the superficial radial ones, that is the three thumb extensors, plus the extensor indicis and some of the extensor digitorum communis tendons to the fingers. Suture of extensor tendons is relatively straightforward and can be carried out in most accident and emergency departments — the technique is described on page 40. If a large number of tendons has been damaged, however, or if the wound is large and irregular, further specialist advice should be sought. The diagnosis of damage to extensor tendons on the dorsum of the wrist and hand is relatively straightforward—a different situation exists distal to the metacarpophalangeal joints, however, as the extensor tendon expands into a broad, thin aponeurotic sheet, and has a number of complicated origins and insertions, whereby the intrinsic and lumbrical muscles effect extension of the inter-phalangeal joints of the fingers. As a general rule, damage to the extensor apparatus of the fingers is best treated with splintage, rather than by open surgery. It is worth repeating that there is nothing to be gained in the casualty department from looking in a lacerated wound at the wrist; the wound should be simply looked at, to gain some sense of its anatomical position, and it should then be covered with a simple dressing and, with the patient relaxed and cooperating, careful estimation of the function of the tendons and nerves distally in the hand and fingers should be made, and it should then be possible to make a reasonably accurate diagnosis of which structures in the wrist have been divided.

THE FRONT OF THE FINGER

Cuts on the front of the finger are very prone to divide flexor tendons and/or digital nerves. This is certainly true of the two proximal phalanges; in the distal phalanx the problem may be better considered as a finger tip injury, which is discussed on page 72. Knowing the instrument causing the wound is most impor-tant—a sharp knife or razor blade will almost certainly have

The Back of the Wrist

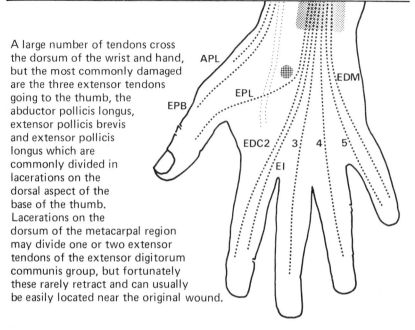

A large number of tendons cross the dorsum of the wrist and hand, but the most commonly damaged are the three extensor tendons going to the thumb, the abductor pollicis longus, extensor pollicis brevis and extensor pollicis longus which are commonly divided in lacerations on the dorsal aspect of the base of the thumb. Lacerations on the dorsum of the metacarpal region may divide one or two extensor tendons of the extensor digitorum communis group, but fortunately these rarely retract and can usually be easily located near the original wound.

The Front of the Finger

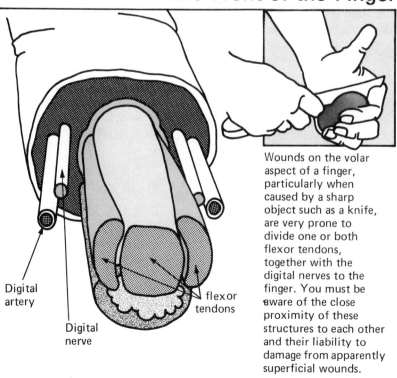

Digital artery

Digital nerve

flexor tendons

Wounds on the volar aspect of a finger, particularly when caused by a sharp object such as a knife, are very prone to divide one or both flexor tendons, together with the digital nerves to the finger. You must be aware of the close proximity of these structures to each other and their liability to damage from apparently superficial wounds.

divided tendons and nerves, whereas a blunter object will be more likely to cause bruising of soft tissues and bony damage. In most situations where a sharp knife damages a finger, the finger tendons are tense as they try to hold the object, and the flexor tendons are therefore brought tight up against the knife with consequent immediate and neat division of the tendons. Digital nerves and vessels lie on either side of the flexor tendon sheath in a smaller fascial compartment of their own, and cannot move out of the way of the knife blade. Division of a digital nerve causes slightly altered sensation in the distal portion of the finger, which can only be detected following a calm examination of a cooperative patient. It is important that these digital nerve injuries should be detected on the day of injury, when repair of the nerves is easily carried out with an excellent prognosis. If the damaged nerve is not appreciated for some time, then repair of a digital nerve after a delay of a week or two can be difficult, and the results are not nearly as good as those following primary repair.

THE BASE OF THE THUMB

Small wounds in this area are often caused by such instruments as a knife which slips, the point of a chisel, or the hand falling on a piece of broken glass. Any wound in this area should be considered as having divided both tendons and nerves until proved otherwise, as it is very easy to miss such damage on a casual examination.

The digital sensory nerves spread out from the median nerve in the base of the palm, and lie a millimetre or so under the skin; the digital nerves to the thumb and index finger can easily be divided via a very small wound. Loss of feeling in the thumb and index finger is a very serious disability, and immediate repair of these digital nerves offers the best chance of recovery of useful sensation.

Slightly deeper to the nerves lie the long flexor tendons to the thumb and index and middle fingers. It is possible to sustain division of digital nerves or tendons alone, but much more common is a combination of tendon and nerve injury, as these structures lie very close together in the palm. A deep wound at the base of the thumb may damage the deep motor branch of the ulnar nerve as it runs across the palm to supply muscles of the thumb/index cleft. It should be possible to diagnose, or at least suspect, damage to the nerve on clinical examination of the adductor pollicis muscle and the first dorsal interosseous muscle and, as with digital nerves, early primary repair of such a small but important nerve is the surest way to regain good function. The diagnosis and treatment of damage to muscles and blood vessels has not been stressed; injured muscles in the hand generally heal perfectly well without specific treatment, and the overall blood supply to the hand is excellent, and there is rarely any need to repair individual divided arteries or veins.

The centre of the palm and base of the thumb is a vitally important area with many significant structures running through it, which are all liable to division from a laceration in this region.

The median nerve in this area is just splitting up into its various branches, both motor and sensory.

The flexor pollicis longus tendon, the two tendons to the index finger and the two tendons to the middle finger are all lying just deep to the median nerve at the base of the thumb.

Deep to the flexor tendons lie the adductor pollicis and first dorsal interosseous muscles with the terminal motor branches of the ulnar nerve running through them. If the laceration is deep enough, this nerve will be damaged with consequent loss of grip in the thumb.

Division of any one of these twelve structures will lead to some significant disability in the hand, and if the laceration is deep enough it is quite possible to divide all twelve of them.

EXAMINATION OF FLEXOR TENDONS

Flexor digitorum profundus

This muscle group has a common muscle mass and splits into four individual tendons which run from the distal forearm through the carpal tunnel out to their insertion in the distal phalanx of each of the four fingers. The index finger profundus tendon is capable of some independent movement, but the remaining three tendons all tend to work together. If the flexor digitorum profundus tendons are intact, then the patient should be able to produce active flexion of the distal interphalangeal joint of each finger. The patient does not need to produce a full range of flexion at the joint, as this may produce some pain in the wound, but if the distal interphalangeal joint is capable of any active flexion, then the profundus tendon is essentially intact.

Flexor pollicis longus

This tendon comes from the same muscle group as the profundus tendons and runs from the distal forearm through the base of the thumb to the distal phalanx of the thumb. The tendon is very liable to damage following cuts on the palmar aspect of the thumb, particularly around the metacarpophalangeal joint. Division of this tendon produces a complete inability to actively flex the interphalangeal joint of the thumb.

Flexor digitorum superficialis

These tendons run superficially through the carpal tunnel, just deep to the median nerve, and spread out to be inserted into the base of the middle phalanx of the four fingers. These tendons flex the proximal interphalangeal joint and their action can be separated from that of flexor digitorum profundus by holding three fingers fully extended then asking the patient to bend the finger in question. With a normally functioning flexor digitorum superficialis, the proximal interphalangeal joint should be capable of easy and strong flexion . . . try it on yourself to appreciate the technique.

Test the flexor digitorum profundus tendon of a finger by holding the metacarpophalangeal and proximal interphalangeal joints extended and have the patient flex the relevant distal interphalangeal joint. He may be reluctant to produce a full range of movement in the joint, due to pain in the wound, but this tendon is the only one which can produce this movement.

The flexor digitorum superficialis tendon may be tested by holding the remaining three fingers extended and have the patient flex the relevant finger. A normal superficial flexor should produce good, strong flexion at this proximal joint, with no *active* flexion occurring at the distal joint.

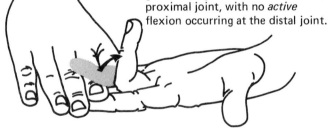

The flexor pollicis longus tendon is tested by holding the metacarpo-phalangeal joint of the thumb extended and having the patient actively flex the interphalangeal joint of the thumb. This is the only tendon which can carry out this action.

EXAMINATION OF EXTENSOR TENDONS

It is rather more difficult to examine the function of extensor tendons via study of the finger joint movement distally, as the extensor tendons do not produce many pure extensor movements of the fingers, and one must take into account the action of the intrinsic muscles of the thumb and fingers on the extensor expansion. The extensor tendons to the thumb, however, if divided, produce an immediate inability to fully extend the metacarpophalangeal and interphalangeal joints of the thumb. With wounds on the back of the hand the finger extensor tendons, if divided, tend not to retract very much because of the intertendonous connections in this area. Damage to extensor tendons on the back of the wrist or hand should be suspected if tendon ends are visible in the wound, or if a patient has difficulty in fully extending the metacarpophalangeal joints of the fingers. A patient with intact extensor tendons should be able to splay his fingers easily and strongly, and indeed the tendons will stand out in the normal hand. Where an extensor tendon has been divided, there is usually a mild, but obvious lag to extension at the metacarpophalangeal joint.

Examination of Extensor Tendons

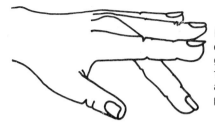

Damage to one of the common extensor tendons to the finger is generally evident as a significant lag to extension when all the fingers are extended at the metacarpo-phalangeal joint.

Loss of either of the extensor tendons to the thumb, but particularly the extensor pollicis longus, is evident as inability to fully straighten the thumb at its interphalangeal joint.

EXTENSOR APPARATUS IN THE FINGERS

Damage to the extensor apparatus of the finger, on the dorsum of the proximal interphalangeal or distal interphalangeal joint generally occurs as the result of a closed injury; the injuries and their treatment are described in this chapter, however, because of the anatomical convenience.

The extensor tendon ceases to be a strong tendonous structure at the metacarpophalangeal joint; as it runs along the dorsum of the finger it thins out into an aponeurotic sheet which is joined at its edges by the small tendons of interosseous and lumbrical muscles. The extensor expansion, as it is now termed, splits into three main bands, a central slip and two lateral bands.

Division or rupture of the central slip, due to trauma over the dorsum of the proximal interphalangeal joint, leads to inability to extend that joint, and if inadequately treated, the full picture of a 'boutonnière' deformity will develop with further lateral slipping of the lateral bands and compensatory hyperextension of the distal interphalangeal joint. With a closed rupture of the central slip, the proximal interphalangeal joint should be splinted in extension, and if there is open division of the slip, it should be carefully repaired *and splinted* in extension. Correct splinting of the proximal interphalangeal joint in this situation may require a properly fitted dynamic splint, and if this is not immediately available, the patient should be referred for orthopaedic or hand surgery opinion.

MALLET FINGER OR 'BASEBALL FINGER'

Sudden, forced flexion of the distal interphalangeal joint, as when the finger is stubbed or when a hand ball is miscaught, may produce a mallet finger deformity – the American term 'baseball finger' is probably a better description. In this injury there is a rupture of the extensor mechanism at the distal interphalangeal joint; the extensor tendon at this level is only a thin sheet of tissue blended with the dorsal joint capsule, and it is relatively weak, certainly when compared with the strong flexor tendon on the palmar aspect of the finger tip. The extensor mechanism may simply tear, but often a fragment of bone is pulled off the dorsal lip of the base of the distal phalanx, although both injuries will produce the same clinical symptoms and deformity; that is an inability to actively extend the distal phalanx.

These injuries, whether soft tissue only, or with a fracture, respond well to simple splintage, keeping the distal interphalangeal joint in the neutral, or slightly hyperextended position, for about 6 weeks. It is important that the patient understands the necessity for the splintage to continue for this period of time. If the splintage is commenced on the day of injury the end result should be good, but if a delay has occurred before seeking treatment, the prospect of recovering a good active range of movement is diminished and orthopaedic referral may be advisable. If the fracture of the distal phalanx involves more than a third of the articular surface of the joint there is a danger that subluxation of the joint may occur, and further advice should be sought regarding the advisability of internal fixation.

Extensor Apparatus in the Fingers

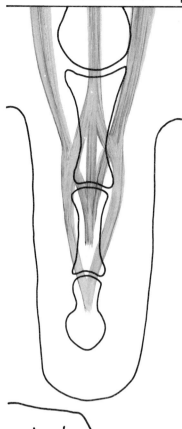

Damage to the extensor tendon, proximal to the metacarpo-phalangeal joint, can be repaired as described on the following page. Distal to the metacarpophalangeal joint, the extensor apparatus ceases to be a tendon and becomes a thin aponeurotic sheet which is less amenable to surgical repair. In general, the proximal or distal interphalangeal joint should be splinted in extension for these types of injury and only rarely should the extensor expansion be sutured.

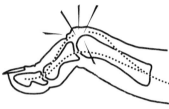

Closed or open ruptures of the extensor mechanism over the dorsum of the proximal interphalangeal joint produce a 'buttonholing' effect, and awkward loss of extension of the joint. These injuries require careful splintage, often with dynamic spring splints, to obtain good recovery.

These mallet or 'baseball' finger deformities should be treated by splinting the distal joint in extension for about 6 weeks, to allow the ruptured tendon to heal without excessive lengthening.

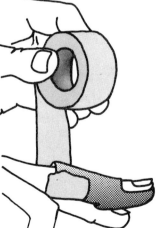

A closed rupture of the extensor mechanism at the distal inter-phalangeal joint—baseball finger—often shows a small fragment of bone avulsed from the distal phalanx on X-ray.

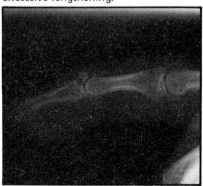

REPAIR OF EXTENSOR TENDONS

When extensor tendons are divided on the dorsum of the hand, in the metacarpal area, they rarely retract, and repair of these tendons is relatively straightforward. Many casualty departments are encouraged to repair these tendons, and providing that good anaesthesia, light, and instruments are available, one should be able to produce a satisfactory result following straightforward repair of the tendons. A careful figure of 8 or 'H' shaped knot, using a suture material of 4/0 (1.5 metric) diameter or stronger, and of a type that you are familiar with handling, should be used. It is important to appreciate that the suture can in no way hold the tendon ends together without appropriate splintage, and indeed the splintage is probably more important than the suturing. All tension must be kept off the suture line by extension of the finger and the wrist, and once the skin has been sutured and a dressing applied, all the fingers of the hand, including the injured one, should be splinted in extension, as should be the wrist. This is best effected by a volar plaster of Paris splint, and should be kept in place for approximately 3 weeks. Thereafter the splint can be shortened to the proximal interphalangeal joint level so that the patient can begin to move his fingers, but the wrist and metacarpophalangeal joints should be kept extended for another 10 days. At the end of a month, extensor tendons are usually well enough healed to allow gentle active mobilisation, but the patient should be kept under review, in case there is any rupture or stretching of the tendon repair.

TREATMENT OF FLEXOR TENDON INJURIES

These injuries are very difficult to treat, and skilled hand surgeons spend a lot of time trying to achieve adequate results following division of these tendons. Any flexor tendon injury must be referred on for specialist advice and treatment. Hand surgeons vary somewhat in their attitude to repair of these tendons, some surgeons preferring to repair all tendons primarily, on the day of injury or soon thereafter, whereas other surgeons prefer to carry out the surgery at a later date, after simple wound toilet and suture of skin only on the day of injury.

From the emergency room point of view, however, it is vitally important that the tendon injury is *diagnosed*, and you must be continually on the lookout for suspicious looking wounds caused by sharp objects on the palmar aspect of the wrist, palm or finger.

Repair of Extensor Tendons

Extensor tendons should be repaired with a simple figure of 8 or 'H' shaped knot, using a strong braided suture which will knot easily.

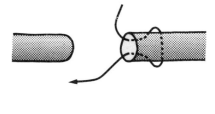

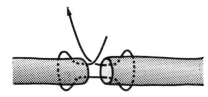
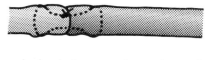

It must be appreciated that this suture is simply to approximate the tendon ends and will not be capable of taking the strain of an actively used tendon. Therefore the tendon must be rested in a splint for some 3 weeks postoperatively. It is not necessary to hold the entire finger extended, but certainly the wrist and metacarpophalangeal joints should be splinted in moderate extension.

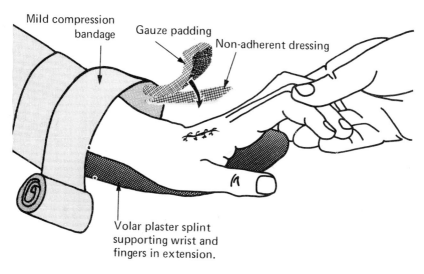

Mild compression bandage

Gauze padding

Non-adherent dressing

Volar plaster splint supporting wrist and fingers in extension.

The treatment of divided flexor tendons is beyond the scope of this book. These injuries must be diagnosed in the accident department, and referred on for treatment by an experienced hand surgeon.

THE MEDIAN NERVE

The median nerve is the most important nerve in the hand because of its sensory supply to the 'business' side of the hand—the thumb, index and middle finger—a hand without sensation here is useless. Division of the digital nerves to the thumb and index finger, which of course are branches of the median nerve, are equally important.

In the forearm, the motor branches of the median nerve supply most of the long flexor muscles of the thumb, index and middle fingers, and usually part of the thenar muscles, that is the short muscles of the thumb. It also supplies one or two lumbrical muscles, but these very small muscles are not capable of examination in an accident and emergency department. Since the median nerve is often cut at the wrist level, the thenar muscles are likely to be partly paralysed, and the one muscle which is regularly supplied by the median nerve is the abductor pollicis brevis. Testing this muscle is straightforward enough, but requires some care with the patient and the manner of testing. Remember the patient probably has a cut wrist and will not be keen on any 'fancy' manoeuvres. Obtain the patient's confidence, that is reassure him, cover up the wound and then persuade him to relax. Gently, starting with the normal side so that the patient understands what is wanted, you position the thumb for him passively in full abduction, and then ask the patient to keep the thumb in this position as you try to push the thumb tip back into abduction, towards the palm. You should in this way be able to feel quite easily the normal abductor pollicis brevis muscle contracting strongly under the skin, if the median nerve is intact. This is a simpler method than persuading scared patients into producing active abduction themselves.

More important, however, is the sensory area of the median nerve. Remember that the thumb, index and middle fingers and the radial half of the ring finger are supplied by the median nerve, although this territory can vary, plus or minus one finger in individual patients. Occasionally patients attend a casualty department and complain of numbness or altered feeling in the hand or finger following a cut in the wrist or palm—more usually, however, the patient is not aware of altered sensation; they are more concerned about the actual cut, the bleeding, the impending sutures etc. and it is your job to reassure them, get them relaxed, and then detect any suspicion of altered sensation. Many textbooks describe an armamentarium of testing pins, bent paper clips, sweat tests and other devices for detecting altered sensation, but in our experience these are out of place in a busy accident department. It is simpler to compare the examiner's finger tip sensation with that of the patient's—he should be able to detect any fine touch between fingers as soon as the fingers touch. If the patient is slow or absent in his response to a simple finger tip touch, then there is likely to be something amiss. The use of a needle or pin is common, but we feel this introduces a further unnecessary object between the examiner and the subject, and furthermore the patient will be apprehensive and expecting pain from a needle, whereas one wants a relaxed cooperative patient if possible.

42

The Median Nerve

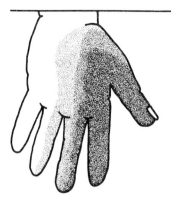

The sensory distribution of the median nerve includes the thumb, index and middle fingers, and the radial half of the ring finger. This area of distribution is not absolute, however, and in some cases of complete median nerve division one may find that only the index finger has apparently deficient sensation.

The only muscle in the hand which is consistently supplied by the median nerve is the abductor pollicis brevis, in the thenar eminence at the base of the thumb. This muscle should be tested by passively putting the patient's thumb in a position of abduction, and then asking him to keep it there, while you, the examining surgeon, attempt to push the thumb back down towards the palm. The patient should be able to resist you, and it should also be possible to feel the short abductor pollicis brevis muscle contracting to hold the thumb abducted if the median nerve is intact.

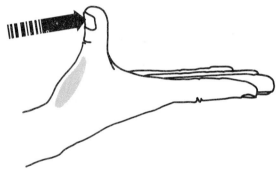

It must be stressed that the median nerve is extremely superficial on the anterior aspect of the wrist and is very prone to damage here. It is most unusual for a patient to actively complain of numbness on the day of injury, and therefore the examining surgeon must treat with suspicion any suggestion of altered sensation associated with a laceration on the front of the wrist or palm.

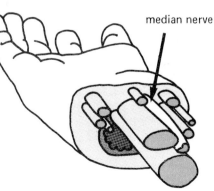

median nerve

THE ULNAR NERVE

This is the main motor supply to the small muscles of the hand—the muscles that produce the wiggly movements of the fingers as opposed to the powerful flexion (median nerve) and extension (radial nerve) of the fingers. After supplying the ulnar portion of the flexor digitorum profundus muscle in the forearm and the flexor carpi ulnaris muscle, it enters the hand in its own tunnel on the ulnar aspect of the wrist and splits into a sensory branch which supplies the skin on the front of the ring and little fingers and a motor branch which supplies the hypothenar muscles and then runs on, deeply, across the palm supplying the interosseous muscles and ending in the adductor pollicis and first dorsal interosseous muscles. Checking sensation in the ulnar nerve is straightforward, using similar methods to those described for the median nerve.

Many tests have been described to assess the motor function in the ulnar nerve, but the following three are straightforward and reliable.

1. Take hold of the patient's index and ring and little fingers with the fingers in the extended position, and ask the patient to move the remaining extended middle finger from side to side. This action requires the action of the volar and dorsal interosseous muscles on either side of the index finger. This movement will be impossible if the ulnar nerve or its deep branch has been divided.

2. With a relaxed patient, and again it is worthwhile starting with a trial run on the normal side to gain their confidence, take the index and little fingers and abduct them, and ask the patient to keep them there as you attempt to close, or adduct, the fingers again. With a separate examining finger, the actively contracting abductor muscles, the abductor digiti minimi, on the little finger, and the first dorsal interosseous on the index finger, can be easily felt – try it on yourself, now.

3. Again with a relaxed patient, move the thumb into adduction, with the first and second metacarpals lying close together, and ask the patient to hold it there as you try to move the thumb away, to open up the thumb/index web as it were. It is not so easy to palpate the adductor pollicis muscle in this situation, but the strength of this muscle is quite obvious if its nerve supply is intact.

RADIAL NERVE

The radial nerve has very little specific function in the hand itself, only supplying a small sensory area of skin on the dorsum of the hand at the base of the thumb. It does, however, supply the motor nerve supply to all the extensor muscles of the forearm, and proximal damage to it, usually above the elbow, results in complete inability to extend the wrist or fingers, giving rise to drop wrist paralysis.

The Ulnar Nerve and Radial Nerve

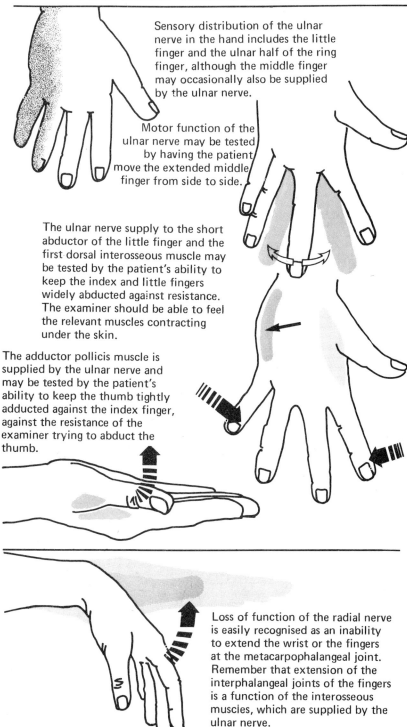

Sensory distribution of the ulnar nerve in the hand includes the little finger and the ulnar half of the ring finger, although the middle finger may occasionally also be supplied by the ulnar nerve.

Motor function of the ulnar nerve may be tested by having the patient move the extended middle finger from side to side.

The ulnar nerve supply to the short abductor of the little finger and the first dorsal interosseous muscle may be tested by the patient's ability to keep the index and little fingers widely abducted against resistance. The examiner should be able to feel the relevant muscles contracting under the skin.

The adductor pollicis muscle is supplied by the ulnar nerve and may be tested by the patient's ability to keep the thumb tightly adducted against the index finger, against the resistance of the examiner trying to abduct the thumb.

Loss of function of the radial nerve is easily recognised as an inability to extend the wrist or the fingers at the metacarpophalangeal joint. Remember that extension of the interphalangeal joints of the fingers is a function of the interosseous muscles, which are supplied by the ulnar nerve.

45

TREATMENT OF DIVIDED NERVES

This section is really about the treatment of *suspected* division of nerves. If there is doubt about the intact function of a nerve, it should be explored; if the nerve turns out to be simply bruised, then the patient is no worse off, the surgeon is reassured; and if the nerve is divided, then a prompt repair can be carried out with the prospect of a good return of function.

All major nerves require exploration and repair in a formal operating theatre with trained staff, good light and fine or micro-instruments. Any suspected damage to the median or ulnar nerve in the wrist or hand should be referred for specialist opinion and treatment.

The following comments apply only to digital nerves in the hand, distal to the midpalmar crease. Many hospitals will prefer to do all nerve repairs, no matter how small, in the operating room with the aid of the microscope, skilled staff, etc., but if these facilities are not available, then it is acceptable to repair small digital nerves in the accident and emergency department. One must, however, have the instruments and skill to be able to handle fine suture material, of the order of 8/0 (0.4 metric) nylon, satisfactorily. A tourniquet must be available to provide a bloodless field, as otherwise dissection and preparation of the nerve is impossible. It is generally necessary to extend the wound, as most wounds in this situation are transverse wounds, and some longitudinal extension of the wound is usually required in order to identify and prepare the nerve ends. It is necessary to separate the nerve from its accompanying artery, and if the artery is divided, both ends should be simply ligated. Repair of the nerve should be carried out using one or two small sutures (fine 8/0 nylon will give a neater and less reactive repair than more traditional materials such as silk, cat gut or human hair).

In a good modern hand surgery unit, a digital nerve would be carefully repaired with very fine nylon under an operating microscope, and the related digital artery, if damaged, would also be repaired. Divided digital nerves are fairly common, however, and most will be seen in an accident and emergency unit without availability of such precise surgery, and if the accident surgeon is capable of using 8/0 nylon, then a satisfactory repair of the digital nerve is certainly worthwhile in that department.

Immediate repair of divided digital nerves is necessary not only to restore sensation in the finger, but also to prevent the formation of painful neuroma at the cut end of the nerve. It is very much easier for the patient and the surgeon to find and repair such small nerves on the day of injury.

Treatment of Divided Nerves

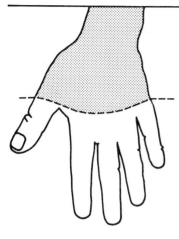

Between the middle of the palm and the proximal interphalangeal joint, digital nerves are relatively easy to find and repair. It is important that these nerves be repaired on the day of injury, as trying to find them and repair them days or weeks later gives an inferior result.

For flexor tendon or digital nerve repair in the hand you need . . .
- *   time
- *   light
- *   instruments
- *   skill

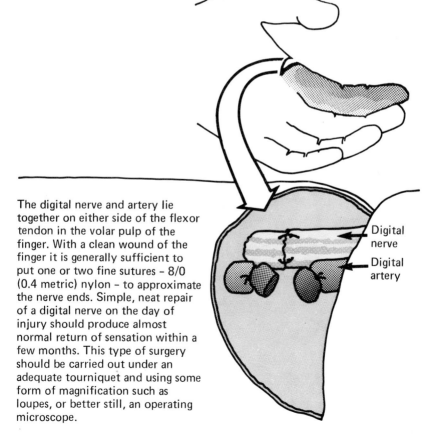

The digital nerve and artery lie together on either side of the flexor tendon in the volar pulp of the finger. With a clean wound of the finger it is generally sufficient to put one or two fine sutures – 8/0 (0.4 metric) nylon – to approximate the nerve ends. Simple, neat repair of a digital nerve on the day of injury should produce almost normal return of sensation within a few months. This type of surgery should be carried out under an adequate tourniquet and using some form of magnification such as loupes, or better still, an operating microscope.

Digital nerve

Digital artery

Chapter 3

LOCAL ANAESTHESIA

The standard solutions used are 0.5, 1 and 2% lignocaine (or Xylocaine, Lidocaine, exactly the same stuff). Use the weaker 0.5% solution for general tissue infiltration and the stronger solution, 1% for blocking nerves; there is rarely any need to use 2% lignocaine in the hand, and it is dangerously easy to inject a toxic dose (10 ml) of the 2% solution.

Long acting agents such as Marcain (bupivicaine 0.25 and 0.5% solutions) can produce nerve block for up to 10 hours, which is useful for long procedures in the arm and hand. Some surgeons feel that the addition of hyalase to local anaesthetic solution will produce a more rapid onset of anaesthesia, particularly in the tight tissue planes on the front of the hand; we have not found this addition to the anaesthetic solution to be necessary for most routine purposes. Beware of using lignocaine with adrenalin (epinephrine)—it is written on the label!—as this can be extremely dangerous in the hand, causing digital artery spasm, and the finger to go black and drop off! The aim of this added adrenalin is to prolong the duration of anaesthesia by reducing the blood flow, but the longer acting solutions such as Marcain will do the job perfectly well. In the majority of minor and straightforward situations in the hand, lignocaine on its own will give perfectly adequate anaesthesia for up to an hour.

Lignocaine is marvellous stuff and if used properly will allow good, painless and confident surgery in the casualty department, *but please give it time to act*—there is no excuse for putting in local anaesthetic and going straight on with the operation—you will scare the patient, hurt him a lot, and put the fear of God into him regarding future local anaesthetics. All local anaesthetics take 10 minutes to act at least, and it is more likely to take 20 minutes if you are trying to block a nerve. Take your time—ideally put in your anaesthetic block and go off and do something else—watch television or whatever, and come back 10 to 15 minutes later and if the local anaesthetic hasn't worked (it usually has), it's your fault; you haven't put it in correctly—it's not the patient's fault if he is rolling around on the bed in pain, it's yours!

Finally, with a nervous or highly strung patient, some additional intravenous or oral Valium is a good and kind idea.

LOCAL INFILTRATION ANAESTHESIA

Local infiltration anaesthesia is easily produced in areas where the tissues are slack, such as the forearm and the dorsum of the hand. Use 0.5 or 1% plain Xylocaine and a fine needle (25 gauge light blue hub). You can either inject from the ends of the wound, making use of the wound itself if it is a clean one, as this avoids piercing the skin, which is usually the most painful part of the procedure. Alternatively, subcutaneous weals may be raised on either side of the wound from a point at either end of it. You should have adequate anaesthesia in 5 minutes, and if the patient still feels pain, remember that it is your fault; you haven't used the lignocaine properly. Some doctors argue that it is not worth putting in local anaesthetic for many lacerations, as the pricks of the injection needle hurt as much as a few quick pricks of the suturing process. You won't find many patients who agree with this philosophy and most suturing procedures usually take longer and are rather more involved than they at first seem, and adequate anaesthesia allows a proper job to be done. Proper treatment of any wound requires adequate cleaning and debridement, exploration and careful suturing, and some of these procedures are very painful unless anaesthetic is used—a large part of your job is to allay the patient's fears and to carry out a calm and efficient diagnosis and treatment without hurting the patient—the proper use of local anaesthesia is vitally important in this.

Remember that local tissue infiltration with anaesthetic solution produces swelling or inflammation following trauma—infiltration is therefore not suitable for areas with tense tissue planes, for example the palm of the hand and the digits. You are generally better off with a proximal nerve block in such areas.

Local Infiltration Anaesthesia

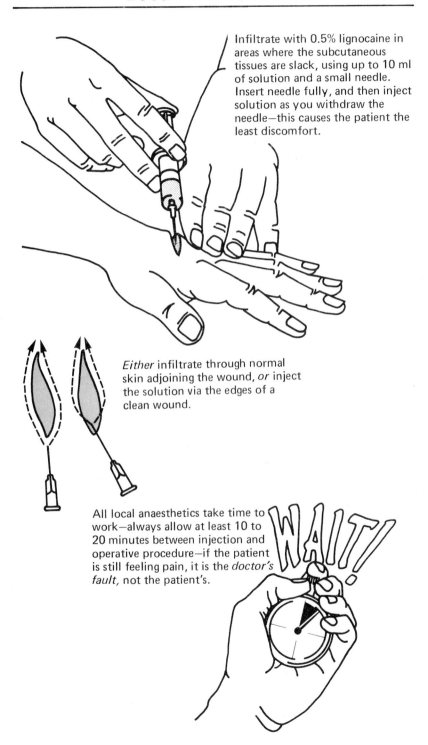

Infiltrate with 0.5% lignocaine in areas where the subcutaneous tissues are slack, using up to 10 ml of solution and a small needle. Insert needle fully, and then inject solution as you withdraw the needle—this causes the patient the least discomfort.

Either infiltrate through normal skin adjoining the wound, *or* inject the solution via the edges of a clean wound.

All local anaesthetics take time to work—always allow at least 10 to 20 minutes between injection and operative procedure—if the patient is still feeling pain, it is the *doctor's fault,* not the patient's.

NERVE BLOCKS—DIGITAL OR RING BLOCKS

This technique is in constant use in casualty departments, and you might as well get it right from the start. The aim is to deposit a volume—2 to 3 ml—of anaesthetic solution, 1% lignocaine, without adrenalin! around the volar digital nerves to the finger. Use a long fine needle (25 gauge, that is a blue hub, is usually best) and insert it on the dorsum of the interdigital web space—the tissues are slack here—and it does not hurt as much as a palmar injection, advance the needle until you meet the palmar skin (from the inside that is) and then inject the anaesthetic as you withdraw the needle; repeat the procedure on the other side of the base of the finger, then make a third injection across the dorsal aspect of the finger in order to catch the fine dorsal digital nerves in this area. Remember—never use solution containing adrenalin (epinephrine) in ring blocks, or indeed anywhere in the hand; a finger may go black and drop off. It is the doctor's responsibility to check exactly what solution he is injecting.

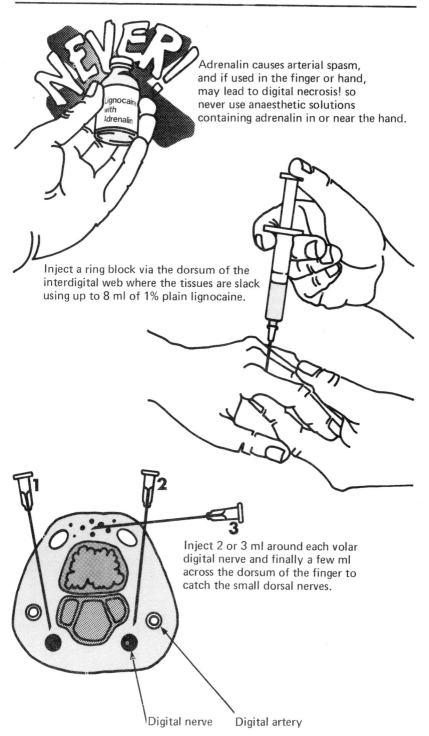

Adrenalin causes arterial spasm, and if used in the finger or hand, may lead to digital necrosis! so never use anaesthetic solutions containing adrenalin in or near the hand.

Inject a ring block via the dorsum of the interdigital web where the tissues are slack using up to 8 ml of 1% plain lignocaine.

Inject 2 or 3 ml around each volar digital nerve and finally a few ml across the dorsum of the finger to catch the small dorsal nerves.

Digital nerve   Digital artery

METACARPAL BLOCK

From time to time there are situations where a block more proximal than the base of the finger is required—for example a laceration or lesion of the web space, and a block of the digital nerves in the metacarpal area may be useful. The digital nerves split up from their parent median and ulnar nerves in the proximal palm and pass distally lying on the lumbrical muscles, between the flexor tendons. It is therefore possible to block the nerves by an injection of 1% plain lignocaine inserted from the dorsum of the hand, between two adjacent metacarpal bones, depositing the solution just deep to (dorsal to) the palmar fascia. If, for example, the middle finger is to be blocked, then an intermetacarpal injection is required between the 2nd and 3rd and 3rd and 4th metacarpals.

BLOCKS OF THE MAJOR NERVES AT WRIST LEVEL

The median, ulnar and radial nerves can all be blocked at wrist level, but the technique is rather more involved than a single ring block, and it takes longer to achieve. Plain lignocaine 1%, 10–15 ml (or 0.5% bupivicaine if a long lasting effect is required) is necessary for each nerve, and should be injected in stages, the initial injection aiming to block the subcutaneous tissues and approximate area of the nerve, while the second portion should aim to deposit solution immediately alongside the nerve. It is best to avoid direct injection into a nerve as this may be followed by long lasting pain and neuralgia from intraneural damage and scarring.

It takes time for anaesthetic solution to diffuse into and through a major nerve, and 20 minutes must be allowed for such a block to take effect.

THE MEDIAN NERVE

The median nerve lies superficially just proximal to the wrist crease, between the flexor carpi radialis and palmaris longus tendons, sometimes lying immediately under the palmaris longus. An initial injection of about 5 ml of 1% plain lignocaine should anaesthetise the skin and subcutaneous tissues, and a second deeper injection of about 8 ml of the same solution will block the tissues immediately adjacent to the nerve. A successful block will anaesthetise the volar aspect of the thumb, index and middle fingers; if the dorsum of the digits is also to be anaesthetised then a separate block of the radial nerve will be necessary.

At least 15 minutes should be allowed for the anaesthetic solution to take effect; if after this interval the patient can still feel pain in the median nerve distribution then a further small injection is required.

Remember, it is not the patient's fault if he is feeling pain, it is yours!

Metacarpal and Median Nerve Block

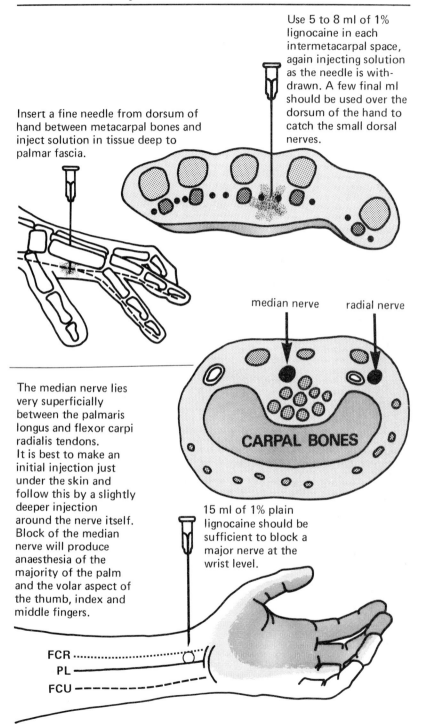

Use 5 to 8 ml of 1% lignocaine in each intermetacarpal space, again injecting solution as the needle is withdrawn. A few final ml should be used over the dorsum of the hand to catch the small dorsal nerves.

Insert a fine needle from dorsum of hand between metacarpal bones and inject solution in tissue deep to palmar fascia.

median nerve   radial nerve

CARPAL BONES

The median nerve lies very superficially between the palmaris longus and flexor carpi radialis tendons. It is best to make an initial injection just under the skin and follow this by a slightly deeper injection around the nerve itself. Block of the median nerve will produce anaesthesia of the majority of the palm and the volar aspect of the thumb, index and middle fingers.

15 ml of 1% plain lignocaine should be sufficient to block a major nerve at the wrist level.

FCR ....
PL ——
FCU — — —

55

THE ULNAR NERVE

The ulnar nerve runs down the forearm to the wrist level, in company with the ulnar artery, lying deep to the flexor carpi ulnaris muscle and tendon. At wrist level, therefore, it can be blocked by an injection just proximal to the wrist crease and between the flexor carpi ulnaris and the palmaris longus tendons. The aim should be to deposit the solution (1% lignocaine or 0.5% bupivicaine, as for the median nerve) in two stages in soft tissues immediately underneath the flexor carpi ulnaris tendon. A successful block will anaesthetise the ulnar portion of the palm and the palmar aspect of the little finger and half of the ring finger. If anaesthesia of the dorsum of these fingers is required, then a further injection around the border of the ulna is necessary in order to catch the dorsal branch of the ulnar nerve, which arises on the main trunk about 8 cm proximal to the wrist and runs dorsally around the ulna.

As with the median nerve, or other major nerve blocks, 15 to 20 minutes is required to allow the anaesthetic solution to penetrate the nerve.

It is also possible to block the ulnar nerve at the elbow, as it is easily palpable just behind the medial epicondyle before it passes deep to the two heads of the flexor carpi ulnaris in the forearm. Once again, the solution should be injected in two phases, initially aiming to block the tissues around the nerve, and the second injection being placed close to the nerve and allowing adequate time for it to take effect.

It is theoretically possible to block the median nerve at the elbow but in practice this is rarely indicated and it is not an easy technique to carry out.

RADIAL NERVE

The radial nerve runs superficially in the subcutaneous tissues of the distal forearm and spreads out over the dorsum of the thumb, index and middle fingers. It is not constant in its anatomical position, so that a specific block of the nerve is not possible, but the area may be anaesthetised by an injection of 8 ml of anaesthetic solution in the subcutaneous tissues around the radial border of the lower end of the radius. All the terminal branches of the radial nerve will be caught by this method, enabling surgical manoeuvres to be carried out on the dorsum of the hand and radial digits.

Ulnar Nerve and Radial Nerve Block

The ulnar nerve at the wrist lies deep to the flexor carpi ulnaris tendon.

FCR ....

PL ——————

FCU – – – – – – –

10 ml of 1% plain lignocaine should be injected deep to the flexor carpi ulnaris tendon—but remember to wait for at least 15 to 20 minutes for the block to work.

Block of the ulnar nerve will produce anaesthesia of the volar aspect of the little finger and the ulnar half of the ring finger. If the block is carried out about 8 cm proximal to the wrist, the dorsal branch of the nerve will be involved in the block and produce anaesthesia of the dorsum of these two fingers.

Ulnar nerve at elbow
It may be more convenient to block the ulnar nerve at the elbow—10 to 15 ml of 1% plain lignocaine should produce anaesthesia of the ulnar one and a half fingers.
Inject the solution between the medial epicondyle and the olecranon, where the nerve can easily be palpated.

Radial nerve
A few ml of 1% lignocaine injected subcutaneously around the radial styloid process will anaesthetise the dorsum of the thumb, index and middle fingers.

AXILLARY BRACHIAL PLEXUS BLOCK

This technique is well worth acquiring for dealing with prolonged or moderately extensive procedures in the hand, wrist and forearm. The success of the injection depends on the anatomical arrangement of the axillary sheath, a tube of dense fascia which encloses the brachial artery and most branches of the brachial plexus as they enter the upper arm. With the patient lying supine, and if he is still at all tense or nervous the use of intravenous Valium may be well-advised, the arm is abducted and externally rotated at the shoulder. It is usually necessary to shave the axilla in order to properly palpate and inject in this area. 30 ml of anaesthetic solution are required, and 1% plain lignocaine will provide fairly rapid onset of anaesthesia which will last for approximately 2 hours. However, if a longer procedure is contemplated, then a 50:50 mixture of 15 ml 0.5% Marcain and 15 ml 1% lignocaine is recommended, as this will produce a long-lasting block for up to 8 house. A fine 23 gauge needle should be used, preferably unmounted initially in order to locate the brachial artery and the sheath, and then the syringe is connected and the solution injected. Palpate the brachial artery high in the axilla, and insert the needle point close to the artery to lie just above or anterior to it—when you let the needle go it should beat up and down with the pulse if you are in the right place. After trial aspiration inject half the solution here and repeat the process immediately below or posterior to the artery. This should ensure that the entire solution has been injected inside the axillary sheath—indeed it is often possible to detect a distinct 'give' in the needle point as you pierce the axillary sheath. A simple rubber tourniquet round the arm distal to the injection site will help to concentrate the solution around the nerves and minimise distal diffusion of the anaesthetic. As a variant of the technique, some prefer to search for paraesthesiae with the needle point; in other words, to find the branches of the plexus more exactly, and while this probably gives more confident anaesthesia, it may alarm the more nervous patient.

SUPRA-CLAVICULAR BRACHIAL PLEXUS BLOCK

This technique will also provide good anaesthesia of the brachial plexus and the whole arm, forearm and hand, but it involves slightly more risk to the patient in that puncture of the apical pleura may produce a pneumo-thorax. For this reason, its use in a casualty department, where the patient is often going home soon afterwards, is not recommended here.

Axillary Brachial Plexus Block

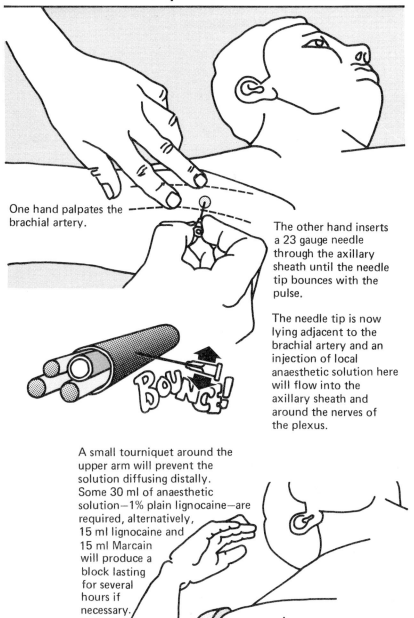

One hand palpates the brachial artery.

The other hand inserts a 23 gauge needle through the axillary sheath until the needle tip bounces with the pulse.

The needle tip is now lying adjacent to the brachial artery and an injection of local anaesthetic solution here will flow into the axillary sheath and around the nerves of the plexus.

Bounce!

A small tourniquet around the upper arm will prevent the solution diffusing distally. Some 30 ml of anaesthetic solution—1% plain lignocaine—are required, alternatively, 15 ml lignocaine and 15 ml Marcain will produce a block lasting for several hours if necessary.

INTRAVENOUS BLOCK (BIER BLOCK)

This is an extremely valuable technique for many procedures in the forearm, wrist and hand, and will produce good anaesthesia for up to 30 minutes. Thereafter the tourniquet cuffs become painful, and while the use of two alternating cuffs will prolong the period of anaesthesia, it is better not to use this method if the surgical procedure is likely to last more than 45 minutes. The principle of the technique is to isolate the circulation of the arm by means of a tight arterial tourniquet, and then fill the venous circulation with a weak solution of lignocaine, which diffuses back into the capillary circulation and produces effective anaesthesia. The patient should be lying down comfortably and, if desirable, a dose of intravenous or intramuscular Valium will help the nervous patient. A good tourniquet with a reliable manometric pressure gauge is required; check that it isn't leaking . . . they often do! A double tourniquet is even better and will enable you to prolong the period of anaesthesia. As a first step after applying the two tourniquets, but before inflating them, insert a small intravenous needle, for example a butterfly variety, into a good vein on the dorsum of the hand. The more distal the vein, the better the anaesthesia. Do not inject anything at this stage, but elevate the arm for a few minutes to drain most of the blood from it—if a particularly bloodless field is required, the hand and forearm should be wrapped up with a soft rubber Esmarch bandage, taking care not to dislodge the intravenous needle. The tourniquet cuff should now be inflated to 300 mm mercury (if two cuffs have been used, inflate the upper, more proximal cuff at this stage)—remember to warn the patient that he is going to feel the cuff tight, but not painful. The arm is now brought down to the horizontal and the Esmarch bandage, if used, removed. Using the intravenous needle, 40 ml of 0.5% plain Xylocaine are injected into the hand and forearm—a mottled appearance of the skin will confirm the area of anaesthesia. As the surgery proceeds, the patient may complain of pain in the area of the tourniquet after 30 minutes or so; if two tourniquets have been used, it is possible to inflate the lower, distal tourniquet, which is now lying over a relatively anaesthetised area, and then deflate the first, proximal tourniquet and this will allow a further period of operating time. When deflating the tourniquet at the end of this procedure it is wise to wait at least ten minutes so that the anaesthetic solution is relatively fixed in the tissues of the forearm, and thereby avoiding a bolus of lignocaine suddenly entering the venous circulation.

Intravenous Regional Anaesthesia

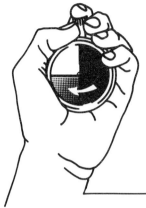

An intravenous block should give 30 min of anaesthesia before the tourniquet cuffs become painful. If two alternating cuffs are used it is possible to prolong the period of anaesthesia to 45 min.

Shopping list—have everything ready before you start!
(1) Butterfly intravenous needle;
(2) strips of adhesive tape;
(3) tourniquet pressure gauge preferably mercury;
(4) two pneumatic tourniquets;
(5) artery forceps to clamp tourniquet tubing;
(6) have ready 40 ml 0.5% lignocaine in 2 X 20 ml syringes.

(a) Apply light tourniquet to emphasise veins;
(b) insert intravenous butterfly needle—as distally as possible and release tourniquet;
(c) elevate arm and/or use an Esmarch tourniquet;
(d) inflate the pneumatic tourniquet on upper arm— inflate the upper tourniquet if two parallel tourniquets are being used;
(e) inject 40 ml of 0.5% lignocaine via butterfly needle;
(f) you should have rapid development of anaesthesia in the forearm and hand, often associated with a mottled appearance of the skin;
(g) at end of procedure deflate tourniquet *slowly.*

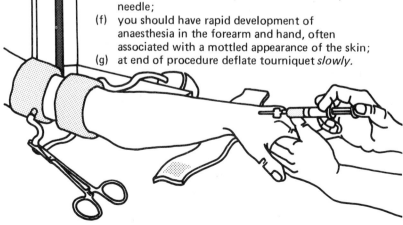

HYALASE

We have not found the use of hyalase, mixed with local anaesthetic, to be necessary in most techniques, but some surgeons prefer using some hyalase in order to produce more rapid spreading of the solution and achieve more rapid onset of anaesthesia.

ETHYL CHLORIDE

This is a painful and rather alarming method of producing mild anaesthesia, and is not used in our department. It is possible to produce some numbness for a very brief period using an ethyl chloride spray, but we feel it is a rather barbarous way of dealing with the patient, and prefer to use lignocaine by infiltration or nerve block.

CONCLUSIONS

Lignocaine is marvellous stuff, and properly used will allow confident and easy surgery without any pain or alarm to the patient. You must know *how* and *where* to inject it, however, and you must *give it time to act*. Beware the use of lignocaine with adrenalin (epinephrine) in the forearm and remember the value of associated Valium or pethidine (Demerol) in nervous patients or when the operative procedure is likely to be long or arduous.

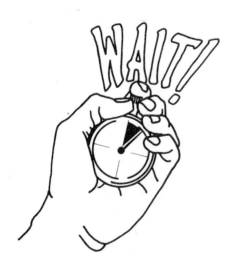

Local Anaesthetic Dosage

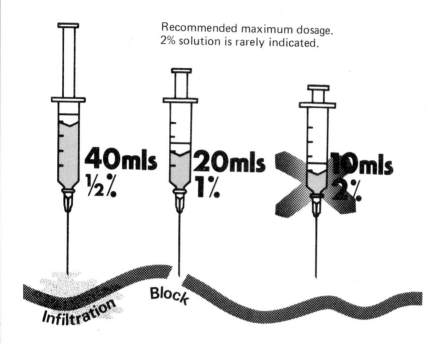

Recommended maximum dosage.
2% solution is rarely indicated.

40mls
½%

20mls
1%

10mls
2%

Infiltration

Block

All patients are nervous and apprehensive—some are very nervous at the thought of an operation no matter how minor. It is well worth administering an intramuscular dose of 10 mg Valium and 50 mg of pethidine (Demerol) (adult dose) 20 minutes before embarking on a surgical procedure.

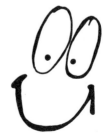

Chapter 4

SUTURES AND DRESSINGS

Clean incised wounds of the hand can, and should be, sutured neatly and precisely in order to achieve good primary healing with minimal scarring. Make quite sure there is no question of tendon or nerve damage in the finger before embarking on a suture in the emergency room, as possible involvement of more vital structures in the finger requires more formal exploration in the operating room.

After appropriate and successful anaesthetic block, the wound should be cleaned, generally with a detergent solution and mild antiseptic solution. If significant or dangerous contamination exists—for example oil injection injury or tooth bites, the wound will need formal exploration and excision in an operating theatre—crushing injuries or other situations where tissue viability is in doubt should also be referred for more formal advice and treatment. An exsanguinating tourniquet is generally helpful in controlling bleeding while the actual suturing is being carried out. If the wound is in the distal half of the finger then a small rubber ring can be used as a tourniquet at the base of the finger, or the finger of a surgical rubber glove can be used, rolled up from the finger tip towards its base, to remove blood from the finger for the duration of the suturing. You must remember, however, if you are using a small tourniquet on the finger, to remove it at the end of the procedure; it is all too easy to leave the tourniquet in place underneath the dressing, and this of course can cause serious damage to the finger. However, if the wound is at the base of the finger, or in the hand itself, then a more proximal tourniquet, preferably of the controlled pneumatic variety on the upper arm will be necessary.

SUTURES AND INSTRUMENTS

A wide range of modern suturing materials and needles are available. Fine monofilament nylon or prolene 4/0, 5/0 or 6/0 (metric equivalents 1.5, 1 and 0.75) on a 15 mm curved cutting needle will produce excellent neat wounds—silk sutures are certainly easy to tie, but produce more tissue and skin reaction in the wound, which lead to a more unsightly scar. Absorbable sutures such as cat gut, Dexon or Tycron, do not require formal removal, but again produce more scar reaction in the wound. It is probably a kindness to use small absorbable sutures in small children, but in adults we feel that fine monofilament nylon is the ideal suture for the skin of the hand.

The handling of fine sutures and needles requires good instruments; often instruments available in the accident and emergency department are far too large and clumsy for good neat suturing of the hand. Fine toothed dissecting forceps of the Adson variety,

A useful finger tourniquet may be made from the finger of a surgical glove, inserted on the finger and then rolled up towards its base. You must, however, *remember to remove* this tourniquet after the procedure is finished.

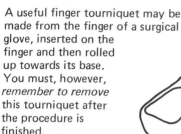

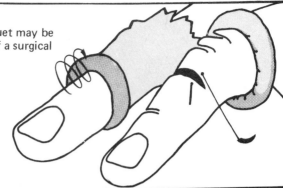

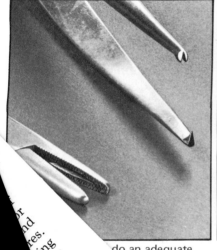

... do an adequate ... ...arse or worn

Fine toothed dissecting forceps and good needle holders with fine, hardened jaws are necessary.

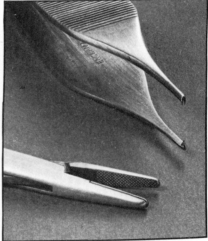

All these sutures are available on a variety of good quality surgical needles, and in general a curved 15 mm cutting needle will be most suitable for skin and an equivalent round bodied needle for soft tissues deep to the skin.

and good needle holders of the Derf or Halsey pattern, approximately 5 in. long, with good tungsten or diamond edged jaws, are necessary. A pair of scissors are also required and these should have long, fine, slightly curved points and the blades should cut well and easily.

SUTURING TECHNIQUE

It is rarely necessary to use subcutaneous sutures in the hand or finger, and the aim is to carefully and neatly approximate the wound edges without tension. All wounds, whether surgical or traumatic, tend to swell slightly for the first day or two, and allowance must be made for this when suturing wounds; it takes some skill and experience to judge the tension when tying sutures so that the final line of the wound heals with a simple, fine scar. It is a common fault for beginners to tie the sutures too tight, and this leads to bunching of the wound and unnecessary scarring. Make a habit of following up the patients and wounds you have sutured in order to check on your own suturing techniques.

To do good suturing of a hand the patient's limb should be well and comfortably supported on a table or arm board, and you, the surgeon, should also be sitting down comfortably with your arms and wrists properly supported. Make sure you have adequate light and that the various instruments, sutures, etc., are within easy reach. Suturing of wounds in the hand can only be done properly using instruments; there is no place for using a hand held needle for this type of surgery. It takes some practice to become adept with these small needle holders; some hand surgeons tend to 'palm' the needle holder as this allows the index finger to lie along the jaws of the instrument, and produces much finer control o[f] the suturing. Straightforward interrupted sutures are ideal f[or] most situations in the hand. Start at one end of the wound a[nd] work steadily along to the other, using fine interrupted sutu[re]. The needle (always use a curved needle with a triangular cu[tting] point) should enter the skin vertically, approximately 2 to [?] from the skin edge and traverse the entire thickness of th[e skin] before emerging horizontally from the subdermal layer. It [is best] to change the needle holder's grip on the needle before pla[cing the] needle in the other side of the wound, and completing th[e suture;] with practice it becomes possible to carry out the sutu[re on both] sides of the wound in one movement.

If the suture material is fine monofilament nylon[, then] it will be necessary to use two or three 'throws' for [the first part] of the knot in order to prevent it slipping, and so th[at the tension] in the knot can be neatly adjusted. One throw [in the opposite] direction to the first will complete the knot; the fi[nished knot should] lie to the side of the suture line as this makes re[moval easier and] allows the surgeon to observe the line of the wo[und]. If interrupted sutures are used with the right te[nsion, the wound] edges will come together neatly without inverti[ng. Careful] adjustment of the wound edge and knot sho[uld prevent] inversion, if persistent, may require the occa[sional mattress suture] to control it. The quality of the skin, its th[ickness]

66

Suturing Techniques

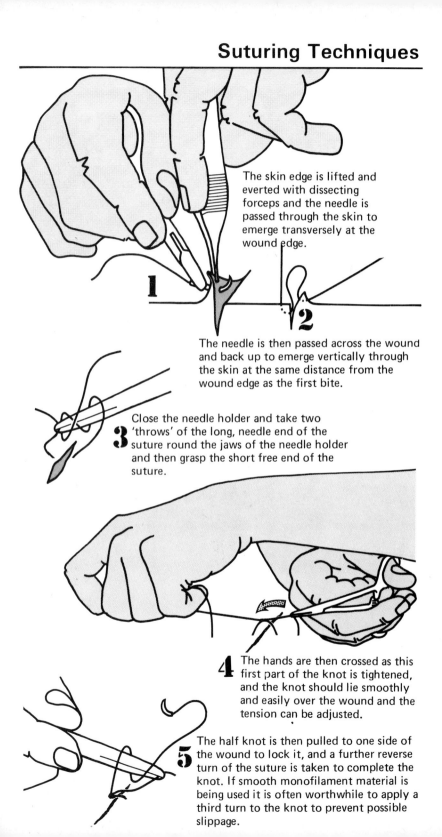

The skin edge is lifted and everted with dissecting forceps and the needle is passed through the skin to emerge transversely at the wound edge.

The needle is then passed across the wound and back up to emerge vertically through the skin at the same distance from the wound edge as the first bite.

Close the needle holder and take two 'throws' of the long, needle end of the suture round the jaws of the needle holder and then grasp the short free end of the suture.

The hands are then crossed as this first part of the knot is tightened, and the knot should lie smoothly and easily over the wound and the tension can be adjusted.

The half knot is then pulled to one side of the wound to lock it, and a further reverse turn of the suture is taken to complete the knot. If smooth monofilament material is being used it is often worthwhile to apply a third turn to the knot to prevent possible slippage.

varies greatly in different parts of the hand and in differing individuals at different ages; it is not possible to define clearly the exact positioning of needles and suture for all situations—only practice and review of your own results will produce a skilled job.

WOUND DRESSING

Dressings on the wound of a hand are important, and it is worth expanding on the aims and methods of a dressing. A dressing applied to a wound in the hand, or indeed anywhere else, is designed to fulfil the following functions:

1. HAEMOSTASIS

Most surgical wounds, no matter how neatly they are sutured, still have a tendency to bleed at the end of a procedure, and this can be minimised or prevented by the careful application of gentle pressure over the whole area of the wound, although if a significant small vessel is still bleeding in the depths of the wound, a dressing cannot control this and re-exploration of the wound will be necessary. Judging the exact amount of tension to apply to a wound is something which only comes with experience, but it should be firm enough to give the patient a feeling of confidence in the wound without causing any pain or embarrassment to the circulation of the finger or hand distally.

2. SUPPORT OF INJURED TISSUES

Normal tissues of the hand, particularly on the palmar aspect, are under some tension, and when the tissue planes are damaged by a wound, this tension is to some degree released. Part of the overall therapy should be restoration of this tissue tension and firmness, and the gentle application of pressure via dressing and bandaging will make the hand feel very much more comfortable and speed the healing process. This application of pressure has to be very carefully done to avoid tight constriction of the bandage proximally which would simply lead to an excess of swelling and oedema in the hand distal to the compressing bandage. Some degree of inflammation and oedema is inevitable after significant crush injuries or burns, but most simple incised wounds should heal satisfactorily without any significant postoperative swelling.

3. SPLINTING THE HAND AND FINGERS

The value of rest in the healing and treatment of wounds in the hand is often under-rated. Any significant wound in the hand will heal very much quicker and more comfortably if the relevant joints are immobilised in a comfortable position. It is generally better to oversplint a hand in the first few days, as this will mini- mise pain and start the healing process. If the whole hand and fingers are splinted in the position of function for a few days, the wound will begin to heal and the patient can then begin to steadily mobilise the finger when the pain and swelling has settled.

Dressing a Wound of the Hand

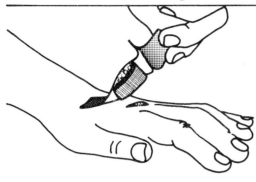

'Band-aid' dressing incorporates all functions of an ideal dressing:
(a) a non-adherent layer next to the wound;
(b) a layer of soft padding, to also absorb exudate;
(c) a firm backing layer which provides splintage and some compression due to its adhesive qualities.

ridged volar plaster of Paris splint to rest and support the hand

further mild compression bandage to support the splinted forearm and hand

mild compression bandage

gauze or wool padding

non-adherent gauze layer

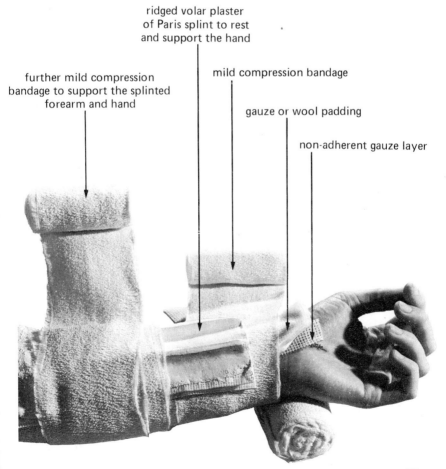

Splinting of the hand need not be absolutely rigid, and we advocate the use of a volar plaster of Paris splint lying superficial to the basic dressing.

4. PREVENTION OF INFECTION

Most wounds are probably secure from external infection a few minutes after the final suture has been tied. Application of an antiseptic layer in a dressing is largely traditional, and it is doubtful whether there is any good case for application of an antimicrobial preparation in the dressing. The most efficient way of preventing infection is to allow the patient's own defences to heal the wound naturally, by providing a neutral wound contact layer such as tulle gras (Xeroform, Jelonet) which also allows easy removal of the dressing. There are certain situations where the use of a medicated tulle gras will be useful, such as a small burn or other open wound where superficial infection is more likely to occur.

5. ABSORPTION OF EXUDATE

Most straightforward wounds do not produce much in the way of bleeding or exudate, but if there has been much tissue damage or if there is any suggestion of infection or burning, then there may well be a considerable amount of serum or other matter which will accumulate in and around the wound and hinder its healing. Surgical gauze is an excellent absorptive layer, although it is easier for the patient and for redressing of the wound later if this absorption occurs through a non-adherent layer such as tulle gras. In certain circumstances where there is a considerable amount of exudate, a more specialised dressing should be used.

6. THE DRESSING SHOULD LOOK AND FEEL GOOD

The psychological effect of a dressing on a hand should not be under-rated; the patient with an injured hand expects to be treated sympathetically and to have kind and efficient therapy with the minimum of pain and fuss. The end point of this process should be the application of a neat and efficient looking dressing which should not be too bulky and should support the hand comfortably. If the patient still has an uncomfortable hand, once the dressing has been applied, then there is probably something wrong.

Dressing a Wound of the Hand

Remember that the bandaged or splinted hand must always lie in the position of function; the wrist should be extended and the thumb should be opposed and able to touch the tips of the index and middle fingers.

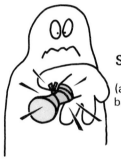

Some common pitfalls of dressings . . . .

(a) beware a tight bandage on a finger;

(b) a finger inside a bandage should be reasonably comfortable; if it continues to be painful, the dressing should be taken off completely and the finger properly examined;

(c) remember that a dressing has to come off after a few days, and the removal of the dressing is often very painful. It is worth obtaining complete haemostasis and dressing the wound carefully with a non-adherent dressing to prevent a painful session at the next dressing clinic.

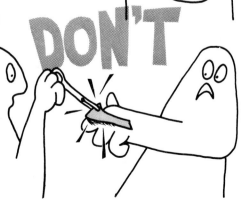

Chapter 5

FINGER TIP INJURIES

AETIOLOGY

Virtually everything we do with our hands involves the finger tips, and it is not surprising that they are injured so frequently. Many such injuries are minor and require simple treatment for a few days only, whereas some apparently minor incidents lead to considerable disability. Some injuries involve damage to the finger tip without actual loss of tissue, whereas other injuries produce loss of skin, pulp, bone, etc. Anyone working in a casualty department should be familiar with the characteristic machinery used in local industry, as the diagnosis, treatment, and rehabilitation of these injuries is often closely related to the type of machinery causing them.

Children are very liable to lose finger tips, often an incomplete amputation, at the toddler stage, from doors shutting on their fingers, and at a rather older age from car doors being slammed or stones and heavy objects being dropped at play. Very sharp objects in the kitchen cause finger tip injuries, usually of a clean slicing variety, carving knives, can openers, broken glass in the kitchen sink. The do-it-yourself workshop and the garden also produce characteristic injuries from electrical circular saws and drills, and from powered grass cutters, particularly the rotary cutting variety.

Industrial injuries range from the straightforward cuts and slices made by butchers' knives, guillotines and ham slicing machines, to the more serious injuries of planing machines, large circular saws, and the crushing injuries associated with heavy steel industries — cranemen, scaffolders, and anyone working in the construction or building industry are very liable to suffer crush fractures of their finger tips. Special attention must be given to any injury caused by a high pressure machine—the injury is *always* much more serious than it appears and usually requires skilled surgical attention. Modern steel presses, injection moulding machines, and particularly high pressure guns of any variety are highly dangerous weapons, and the injuries they cause must be treated with extreme care. (High pressure injection injuries are dealt with under the heading of Foreign Bodies, page 90).

Remember that the finger tip is an extremely sensitive area and that these injuries, in some ways minor injuries, are generally very painful; it is not uncommon for patients to be off work for a year or more due to inappropriate initial treatment for an apparently minor finger tip injury. Patients should be followed up for the first few weeks to ensure that the wound heals promptly and neatly and that the patient is able to return to work without delay.

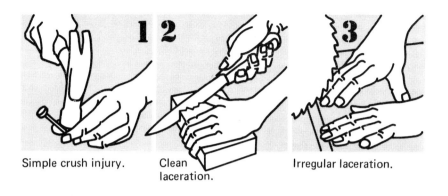

Simple crush injury.

Clean laceration.

Irregular laceration.

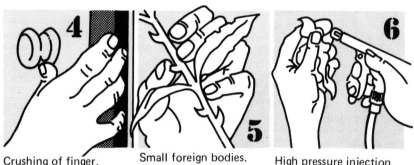

Crushing of finger, especially in children.

Small foreign bodies.

High pressure injection injuries.

ANATOMY

The tips of the fingers are vitally important and very delicate sense organs. The skin and pulp of the distal phalanx is packed with nerve endings and any injury to this area is extremely painful and any loss of function due to nerves, skin or sensitive scarring can make the finger useless. Many problems of disability in the hand are caused by failure to appreciate the importance of the various parts of the finger tip, or to inadequate treatment of finger tip injuries. The skin of the volar surface of the distal phalanx is much thicker than normal skin and has a particularly abundant sensory nerve supply –this area is one of the more sensitive in the body and the two point discrimination here is of the order of 2 to 3 mm (forearm 20 mm, skin of the back 60 mm). Sweat glands exist in abundance, and the skin is thrown into characteristic folds producing the individual finger prints. The skin is supported by the pulp of the finger tip which is a tough fibro-fatty tissue attached to the tuft of bone at the tip of the distal phalanx; this pulp is extremely important in giving the skin the necessary padding and support for adequate gripping and feeling. Through the pulp run the arteries and digital nerves to supply the finger and the finger tip. In the deepest part of the pulp the flexor tendons run in their fibrous sheath, the profundus tendon ending at its insertion into the front of the distal phalanx. The skeleton of the distal phalanx is securely attached to the skin of the finger tip by strong fibrous tissue strands, which run from the skin through the pulp to the bone. This relationship of skin, pulp and skeleton exists over the entire palmar aspect of the fingers and palm of the hand, resulting in a high pressure system, and any increase in pressure on the volar aspect, such as an abscess, is particularly painful, although there may be very little swelling on the anterior aspects of the hand; any swelling tends to occur on the dorsal aspect of the finger or hand, where the tissues are much slacker, this being the low pressure area of the hand where the venous drainage occurs.

On the dorsum of the finger tip the finger nail lies on the nail bed, the proximal portion of which is the germinal zone or lunula, which shines through the finger tip as a white crescent. It is this germinal zone which produces the actual growth of the nail and the nail is then supported distally on the nail bed until it runs free over the tip of the finger. Damage to the finger nail does not affect the function of the finger as much as damage to the pulp, but the disfiguring effect is considerable and damage to the finger nail or nail bed may give rise to recurrent problems of infection and deformed growth of the nail.

74

Anatomy of the Finger Tip

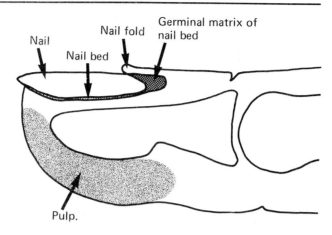

Nail

Nail bed

Nail fold

Germinal matrix of nail bed

Pulp.

It is important to appreciate that the pulp of the finger tip with its overlying skin is a very delicate and sensitive organ. Damage to the pulp or the skin of the finger tip is disabling for that digit, and if the wound does not heal properly, then the patient avoids using the finger, and the hand as a whole is at a disadvantage for many tasks and functions.

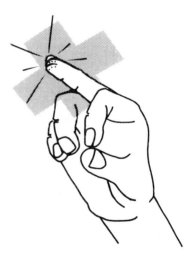

CONCEPTS OF TREATMENT

When faced with a finger tip injury, it is important to decide whether there has been any significant tissue loss, as this will dictate the lines upon which treatment will be carried out. Concepts of treatment are worth considering under the following headings:

> No tissue loss;
> Loss of skin only;
> Loss of skin and pulp;
> Loss of skin, pulp and bone.

NO TISSUE LOSS

Where the wound is a straightforward crushing injury or simple laceration, no tissue will have been lost, and treatment consists of cleaning the finger tip, careful suturing of any wounds and appropriate splintage or other method to make the finger comfortable. The first step of treatment should be the production of an effective anaesthetic block of the finger, best done by means of a ring block at the base of the finger. Once the finger is anaesthetised, the injury can then be properly assessed and cleaned, and any debris or haematoma removed. If a haematoma exists underneath the nail, this can be released simply by drilling a small hole in the nail, or burning a hole with a heated end of a paper clip. Skin wounds should be sutured using the finest suturing material that you can usefully handle, preferably 5/0 or 6/0 (1 and 0.7 metric) nylon, and the neater the job you do initially, the better will be the end result, both from the point of view of function and appearance. Injuries to the nail and nail bed are often underestimated, and a laceration or tear of the nail bed should be treated exactly as a tear in the skin, that is by careful repair with a fine suture material. It is generally necessary to remove the nail in order to assess the damage to the nail bed properly, but if the repair is done effectively on the day of injury, it will prevent later scarring and deformity of the nail. A small piece of tulle gras (Xeroform) should be inserted under the nail fold after removal of a finger nail, in order to prevent adhesions occurring between the fold and the nail bed, which in turn will impede the growth of the new nail.

Crush injuries of the finger tip are generally associated with undisplaced comminuted fractures of the distal phalanx, and these fractures require no specific treatment, apart from releasing tense haematoma and gentle splinting of the finger. In a strict theoretical sense, crush fractures of the distal phalanx are compound fractures, but the formal routine of excision of wound edges, full cleansing of the wound and the fracture site, and intensive antibiotic therapy, which one would carry out for a compound fracture of a major long bone, would be wasteful overtreatment for these essentially minor injuries.

Finger Tip Injuries

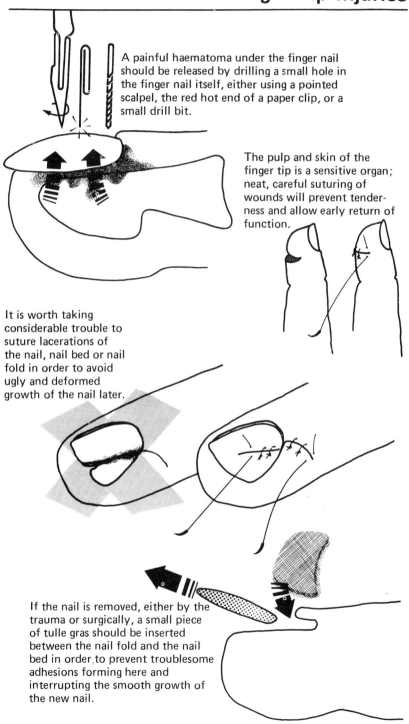

A painful haematoma under the finger nail should be released by drilling a small hole in the finger nail itself, either using a pointed scalpel, the red hot end of a paper clip, or a small drill bit.

The pulp and skin of the finger tip is a sensitive organ; neat, careful suturing of wounds will prevent tenderness and allow early return of function.

It is worth taking considerable trouble to suture lacerations of the nail, nail bed or nail fold in order to avoid ugly and deformed growth of the nail later.

If the nail is removed, either by the trauma or surgically, a small piece of tulle gras should be inserted between the nail fold and the nail bed in order to prevent troublesome adhesions forming here and interrupting the smooth growth of the new nail.

LOSS OF SKIN

Where children are concerned, the loss of skin or even skin *and* pulp from the finger tip will often heal remarkably well following straightforward cleaning and re-dressing of the finger at intervals over a few weeks. The child's tissues have remarkable powers of regeneration, and it is rarely necessary to become involved in complicated surgical techniques.

The adult finger tip, however, does not repair so well, and if an area of skin greater than 1 cm in diameter has been lost, then consideration should be given to replacing this area with a free skin graft. This is not a complicated procedure and with a little practice a skin graft can be taken using a large scalpel blade or a small Silver skin grafting knife which takes a small razor blade. The anterior aspect of the forearm is commonly used as a donor site, but a better area in many ways is the ulnar border of the hand, where the skin is of similar thick quality to that of the injured finger tip, and the donor site here heals without any trouble. It is vitally important that all bleeding should have ceased from the wound of the finger tip before the skin graft is applied, and the graft should then be sutured in place with fine sutures, perhaps reinforced with adhesive paper tape. It may be helpful to apply a small tie-over dressing (stent) using the long ends of the sutures to produce some gentle compression over the skin graft, and thereby prevent the accumulation of haematoma under the graft. The finger should be very thoroughly splinted after this type of procedure, and it is best to splint the neighbouring fingers also, and instruct the patient to keep the hand and arm well elevated for the next 24 hours to prevent the risk of bleeding under the graft.

It may occasionally be more convenient to remove the graft on the day of injury, but simply store it in the refrigerator, soaked in sterile saline, with the patient's name clearly on the bottle, and then apply the skin graft a week later when the original wound has begun to form clean red granulation tissue, and the skin graft will then take easily.

It takes a little experience to judge the thickness of skin grafts correctly, but as a general rule you should leave the donor site with a few little spots of blood coming through the dermis, and if you can see fat on the under surface of the skin graft, then you've taken it a bit too thick, as this implies you have taken the full thickness of skin, rather than ideal partial thickness graft. In general, the thinner the skin graft, the easier it will 'take', but the less hard wearing it will be, and it will also tend to contract more. A thicker split skin graft, however, is much more durable, but may not 'take' quite so easily and you therefore have to take careful precautions to prevent haematoma formation underneath the graft or any tendency for the graft to move around on the recipient site.

Finger Tip Injuries – Skin Grafting

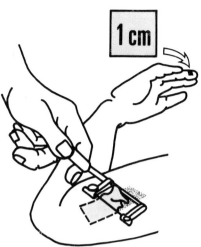

Small split skin grafts for use on the hand may be conveniently removed from the medial aspect of the forearm or upper arm by means of a small Silver skin knife, which uses standard razor blades. The area to be used as the donor site should be anaesthetised with subcutaneous 0.5% lignocaine plus adrenalin (epinephrine), which outlines the area that is anaesthetised and reduces the bleeding.

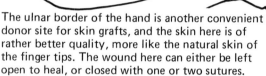

The ulnar border of the hand is another convenient donor site for skin grafts, and the skin here is of rather better quality, more like the natural skin of the finger tips. The wound here can either be left open to heal, or closed with one or two sutures.

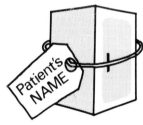

If you end up with too much donor skin, or if it is inconvenient to apply the skin graft immediately, it is possible to store split skin grafts for up to 3 weeks, if it is kept moist in a securely closed sterile container in a refrigerator at 4°C. Make sure that the container is clearly labelled with the patient's name, the date and the surgical unit.

It is important that a split skin graft is gently, but firmly attached to the wound, particularly to avoid slippage, or haematoma formation in the first few post-operative days. A number of fine sutures around the periphery of the graft, with their ends left long and tied over a small moist dressing, or stent, is the most reliable way of achieving a good 'take'.

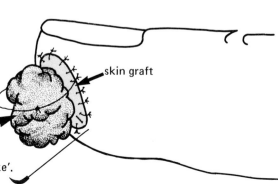

skin graft

LOSS OF SKIN AND PULP

When a significant amount of the *pulp* of the finger tip has been lost with the skin of the finger tip, the problem becomes more complicated. Placing a skin graft, or other repair, over the bone of the distal phalanx without the important padding layer of the pulp will result in a thin, tender and painful finger tip which is useless for any practical purposes. Various surgical manoeuvres are available to produce a well contoured finger tip, with an adequate, almost normal pulp; these techniques are somewhat small and tricky however, and you must bear in mind that you should be advising the neatest and simplest treatment that you are capable of carrying out confidently, with the aim of having the finger back in use, and the patient at work, in about 3 weeks.

Small children often remove, completely or partially, the skin and pulp of a finger tip in the door of a house or car. It is well worth suturing these composite tissues back in place—after appropriate anaesthesia and cleaning—as they will generally survive and result in a virtually normal finger tip. Even if the amputated finger tip is missing it may well be best to simply clean and dress the wound, allowing it to heal naturally, as small children's fingers have a remarkable ability to regenerate lost pulp and skin.

In the adult situation however, the loss of skin and pulp presents considerable problems, as replacing the skin, without the pulp, is liable to produce a thin scarred finger tip, too tender for routine work.

If the angle of the wound is vertical or angled dorsally it may be

advisable to move a small local flap of skin and pulp from the volar aspect of the finger (a V–Y advancement) to cover the defect at the tip. This however is a rather tricky procedure and advice should be sought from a plastic or hand surgeon. A simpler solution would be to nibble away a little of the bone of the distal phalanx, thereby shortening the finger tip, but allowing easy closure of the skin edges.

If the wound is angled to the volar aspect there will be considerable loss of pulp, and in this situation some form of pedicle flap, such as a cross finger flap, will be necessary, or the patient will have to accept some considerable shortening of the finger. Such shortening of the finger—terminalisation— 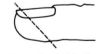 may well be the best solution in a manual worker, but if the patient wishes to retain the length and appearance of the finger a second opinion should be sought regarding a composite flap to replace missing pulp and skin.

The selection of the best repair for any particular finger tip injury can be difficult—a young female musician will require an entirely different repair from a middle-aged construction worker— and it is generally best to seek advice from a plastic or hand surgeon before embarking on ambitious surgery.

Finger Tip Injuries – Tissue Loss

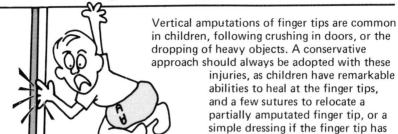

Vertical amputations of finger tips are common in children, following crushing in doors, or the dropping of heavy objects. A conservative approach should always be adopted with these injuries, as children have remarkable abilities to heal at the finger tips, and a few sutures to relocate a partially amputated finger tip, or a simple dressing if the finger tip has been completely lost, will generally produce a very worthwhile result.

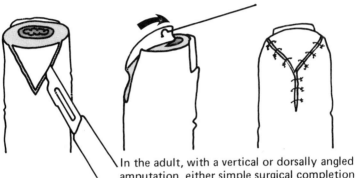

In the adult, with a vertical or dorsally angled amputation, either simple surgical completion of the amputation, or cover of the tip of bone by moving a small triangle of skin and pulp distally should be considered. This latter procedure is very neat, but requires careful judgement and skill to succeed, and if in doubt the opinion of a hand or plastic surgeon should be sought.

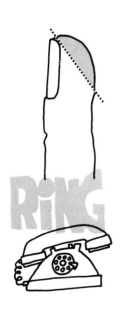

Where the amputation of the finger tip involves loss of the volar tissue, the skin and pulp of the finger, the choice of treatment will lie between completing the amputation by shortening the finger tip by a few cm. or replacing the lost skin and pulp by means of a pedicle flap. A variety of pedicle flaps can be used in the hand, but for this particular injury, a cross finger flap is probably most convenient, but this does require relative skill and experience in turning flaps and it is best to ask for help from a hand or plastic surgeon in this situation.

Chapter 6

AMPUTATIONS

If the finger tip is so badly damaged that shortening of the finger is necessary, the surgery should be carried out in a positive fashion with the aim of giving the patient a well healed, non-tender stump with a good range of movement in the remaining joints.

The temptation to preserve length in the fingers must be resisted; of far more importance is the creation of a slack suture line, with no digital nerve remnants involved, otherwise a tight, painful and tender stump will result. Loss of the distal phalanx of a finger or indeed the distal two phalanges of a finger, will cause remarkably little disability, assuming the resulting stump is not tender or painful. The thumb poses a special problem, and although shortening to the level of the interphalangeal joint causes little disability, if the damage to the thumb implies an amputation through the proximal phalanx, or more proximal than this, then further advice should be sought—there are a number of procedures available for preserving or recovering length in a short thumb, but these require advanced plastic or bone procedures.

With fingers damaged more proximally, the aim should be to provide comfortable wound closure rather than maximum length.

In the index finger, a stump shorter than the proximal interphalangeal joint level is unlikely to be of much use in gripping, and a complete ray resection, that is removing the finger through the proximal third of the second metacarpal, will produce a better looking hand than one with an awkwardly short and useless stump of proximal phalanx.

When amputation of one of the central digits, the middle or ring finger, is necessary, it is worthwhile preserving even a short stump of proximal phalanx, as the cosmetic defect is often slight, especially when the hand is viewed from the dorsal aspect, and also the cupping effect of the hand is preserved. Patients who have lost a complete middle or ring finger will complain of losing coins through the gap in their hand!

With amputation of the little finger the patient's occupation is important—anyone who uses tools and requires a strong power grip will value a portion of the proximal phalanx of the little finger, whereas a woman may prefer the less unsightly appearance of a ray resection through the shaft of the 5th metacarpal bone.

Amputation: Problem Zones

A well-healed, comfortable finger amputation is much more important than a few cm extra length.

Amputations in the proximal half of the thumb may require complex reconstructive techniques, and further advice from a hand surgeon should be sought.

In the distal half of the thumb, the aim should be to achieve good primary healing rather than strive to maintain length.

Most patients with damage to the proximal half of the index finger will be better off with a complete ray resection.

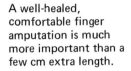

If the base of the little finger is damaged, however, a ray resection to the base of the 5th metacarpal will produce a more acceptable cosmetic result.

In the middle and ring fingers it is worth preserving even a small stump of the proximal phalanx, as this improves the appearance of the hand, and preserves the cup type of grasp.

The base of the proximal phalanx should be preserved, particularly in men doing heavy work, as this is very useful for controlling tools.

Obtain good primary healing in the distal half of the fingers.

The comments on this page refer only to single digit amputations; where more than one digit has been damaged, further advice from a hand surgeon should be sought.

TECHNIQUE OF FINGER AMPUTATION

A local anaesthetic block at the base of the finger, aided by a small rubber tourniquet or finger of a surgical glove, to control bleeding (see page 64), should provide excellent conditions for minor amputation surgery. After removing all damaged skin, subcutaneous tissue and bone, the dorsum of the finger should be examined to ensure that no nail bed remnants remain—excise the soft tissue right down to the bone in this area, so that there is no chance of the nail re-growing and causing later problems in the amputation stump. Establish the length and shape of the skin flaps—ideally producing a larger volar flap than a dorsal one, so that the eventual scar lies dorsally, and the volar aspect of the stump will then be covered by good volar pulp and skin. The bone of the finger should now be shortened so that the skin flaps will close *easily* over the bone ends without tension—this is probably the commonest cause of unsatisfactory amputation stumps in inexperienced hands.

If the level of section falls through a joint, it may be worthwhile to trim the edges of the condyles of the phalanx to avoid too bulky a stump, but there is no need to remove the cartilage from the head of the phalanx. The extensor tendon is simply transected at the same level as the bone, and the flexor tendon, or tendons, should be simply transected at the level of bone division, and a suture through the tendon and tendon sheath will encourage adhesions at this level, thereby providing some additional flexion power in the amputated finger.

The neurovascular bundles, one on each side of the finger, must be dissected carefully and each artery ligated and the digital nerve shortened. It is extremely important to find the digital nerves and ensure that the severed ends lie well clear of the terminal amputation scar in the finger. A number of sophisticated techniques for dealing with the digital nerve end have been described, but we find that simple division and/or ligature of the nerve end and allowing it to retract into the stump, gives excellent results in primary amputation.

Final suture of the skin requires neat approximation of the flaps with fine nylon, using interrupted sutures and with no tension in the wound edges. Make sure the proximal tourniquet, if used, has been released and that the stump wound has stopped bleeding before applying a final dressing.

Remember that two common problems following amputation of a finger are an excessively tight and tender stump due to the skin being too thin and tight over the end of the bone, and tender neuroma formation from the end of the digital nerve being adherent to the terminal scar. Both these problems can be avoided by careful attention to operative technique.

Technique of Finger Amputation

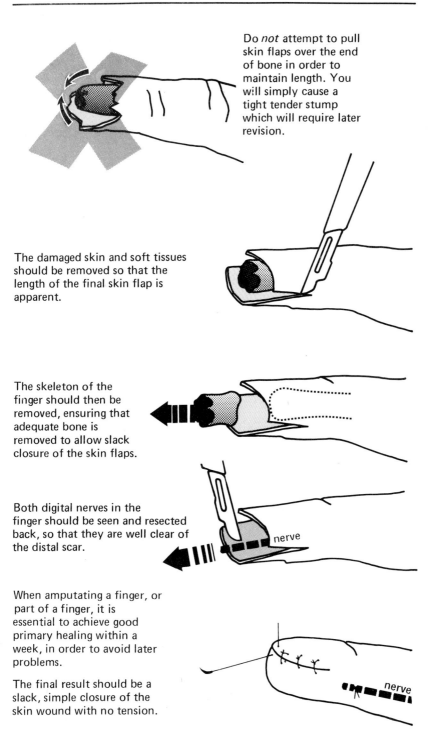

Do *not* attempt to pull skin flaps over the end of bone in order to maintain length. You will simply cause a tight tender stump which will require later revision.

The damaged skin and soft tissues should be removed so that the length of the final skin flap is apparent.

The skeleton of the finger should then be removed, ensuring that adequate bone is removed to allow slack closure of the skin flaps.

Both digital nerves in the finger should be seen and resected back, so that they are well clear of the distal scar.

nerve

When amputating a finger, or part of a finger, it is essential to achieve good primary healing within a week, in order to avoid later problems.

The final result should be a slack, simple closure of the skin wound with no tension.

nerve

REPLANTATION

Modern microsurgery, as practised in certain centres, permits replantation of completely severed hands, fingers or even portions of fingers. The techniques are complex however, and only parts which have been severed in a clean fashion by a sharp blade or instrument will produce a worthwhile result. The amputated part should be of significant value to the patient—for example an amputated little finger is best accepted, whereas an amputated thumb or major portion of the hand should certainly be considered for replantation. It is important that time should not be wasted, and in order to prolong the survival time of the amputated part, it should be cooled, preferably by placing it in a clean plastic bag, placing this bag inside a second plastic bag containing ice. The patient should be reassured and standard resuscitation methods carried out—although patients with a clean cut amputation often lose surprisingly little blood—and the nearest microsurgical unit should be contacted. If you don't know where the nearest unit is, get on the telephone promptly and find out.

Replantation of Amputated Digit

A cleanly amputated hand or digit can be replanted using modern microsurgical techniques in the hand or plastic surgery unit.

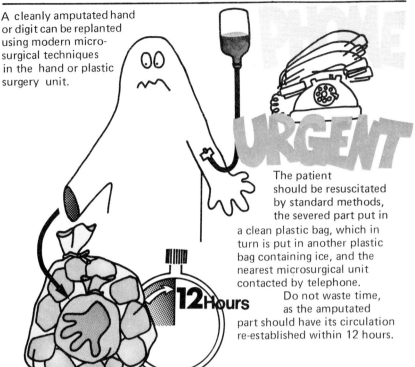

The patient should be resuscitated by standard methods, the severed part put in a clean plastic bag, which in turn is put in another plastic bag containing ice, and the nearest microsurgical unit contacted by telephone. Do not waste time, as the amputated part should have its circulation re-established within 12 hours.

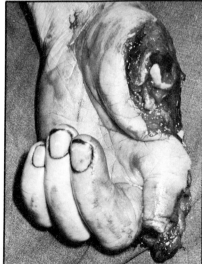

Traumatic amputation of left thumb and index finger.

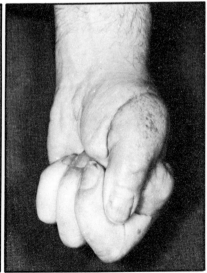

Left thumb following successful replantation; the index finger was badly damaged and was not replanted.

Chapter 7

FOREIGN BODIES

The hand is a common site for foreign body injuries. If the patient has a recent wound and a radio opacity on X-ray, the diagnosis is obvious; often, however, there may be no wound, or an extremely small one, or it may have already healed—if you have any suspicions at all, have the hand X-rayed, preferably with soft tissue penetration to show up any mildly opaque materials such as wood or glass.

In the acute situation, if the foreign body is very superficial or can be seen in the wound, it should be removed. If the material has been implanted for some time, or if it is deep to the subcutaneous tissue, it is much wiser to refer the patient for an elective exploration of the hand with full operating theatre facilities. Much harm can be done by inexperienced attempts at dissection in the hand in a casualty department, where full hand operating facilities are not available.

NON-IRRITANT FOREIGN BODIES

These are generally sharp, broken ends of brittle objects, such as sewing needles, wood splinters, flakes of steel from chisels or hammers, and fragments of glass. Once the diagnosis has been established—and an X-ray *must* be taken—the fragment should only be removed if it is manifestly superficial and easy to get at. It is often better to simply close the wound and refer the patient for formal exploration of the wound some weeks later. These foreign bodies rarely cause significant symptoms, and at a delayed operation a capsule has usually formed around the object and this makes finding and extracting it very much easier. Because many of these objects are sharp at one end only they often travel through the tissues and an immediate preoperative X-ray should be taken to establish the current position of the object. Foreign bodies under a finger nail, generally a splinter of wood, can be difficult to remove, and the patient has generally tried to remove it himself without success. Following an adequate anaesthetic block of the finger, a simple wedge of nail can be excised over the splinter and it is then easily lifted out.

IRRITANT FOREIGN BODIES

A number of vegetable and animal thorns are capable of producing considerable irritation in the hand, and the patient often presents some time after the injury with a painful or swollen finger or hand. Thorns, cactus and sea urchin spines, are all capable of this irritation, and careful exploration of the skin and subcutaneous tissues is generally required to cure the problem. Some such thorns and spines may present as frank abscesses, and on drainage of the cavity the foreign material is discharged with the pus.

88

Foreign Bodies in the Hand

Do *not* fiddle around in a wound of the hand trying to locate a foreign body. You are unlikely to find the object, and you are very likely to do damage to nerves, tendons and other structures in the hand.

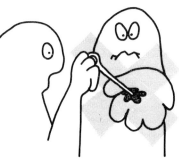

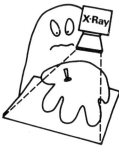

The hand should be X-rayed to locate the foreign body. Foreign bodies are all radio-opaque to some degree, even wood or glass.

The common problem of a splinter of wood under the finger nail is best dealt with by local anaesthetic block of the finger and excision of a wedge of nail over the splinter when it can easily be removed.

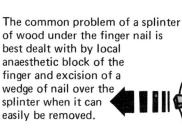

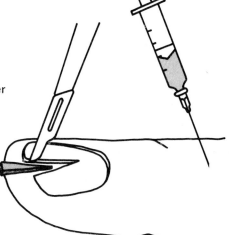

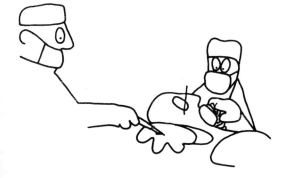

It is often more convenient to leave a small foreign body in the hand, allow the entry wound to heal, and then remove the foreign body at a later date, if it is causing trouble, at an elective operation with proper operating theatre facilities.

HIGH PRESSURE INJECTION INJURIES

These injuries are always serious, and must be promptly treated by an experienced hand surgeon. It is vitally important for the casualty staff to recognise and diagnose this type of injury, hence one must always determine what type of machine caused the injury. Many modern engineering and painting processes make use of high pressure injection guns, and it is all too easy for the operator to inject a few millilitres of fluid into his hand, usually the non-dominant index finger, as it is used to wipe excess paint, grease or oil from the gun nozzle. Often there is no detectable entry wound, and indeed the patient may not be aware of the cause of his symptoms—any painful or swollen finger in a patient who works with high pressure guns must be presumed to have injected foreign material into the hand.

It is important to realise that the few millilitres of noxious fluid injected into the finger tip instantaneously travel up the finger to the palm of the hand, often in the flexor tendon sheath, and set up an intense chemical inflammation. If treatment is delayed, the patient will probably lose the finger, and possibly part of the hand. Do not waste time, but contact a hand surgery unit for immediate exploration of the finger and hand.

With thick oil and grease it is possible to remove most of the material, but paints and volatile organic solvents tend to vaporise rapidly in the finger and cause widespread and intense necrosis and inflammation.

High Pressure Injection Injuries

These are very dangerous injuries and may lead to the loss of a finger or part of the hand. The initial wound may seem trivial and unimportant, but it is vitally important to determine which type of high pressure machine or gun caused the injury.

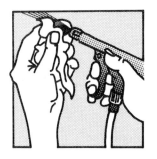

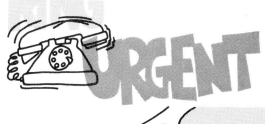

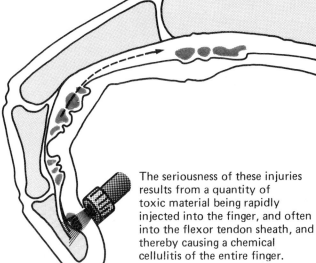

The seriousness of these injuries results from a quantity of toxic material being rapidly injected into the finger, and often into the flexor tendon sheath, and thereby causing a chemical cellulitis of the entire finger.

The standard treatment of these injuries is *immediate* exploration of the finger by a competent hand surgeon and thorough cleansing of all affected tissue.

Chapter 8

INFECTION

The patterns of infection in the hand have changed dramatically over the past 20 years, and while the majority of hand infections are now relatively minor affairs, the occasional palmar abscess or spreading infection is a reminder of how serious the complications of hand infection can be. Despite the large variety of initiating wounds, the infecting organism in hand infections is remarkably consistent; the *Staphylococcus aureus*, generally penicillin resistant, is found in over 95% of hand infections. While the initial inoculum of bacteria may contain a wide range of bacteria, the *Staphylococcus aureus* soon predominates and produces the classical abscess containing yellow pus.

Infection can be introduced to the hand via a wound in any site, but the most common area for an initial infection is the finger tip, including the finger nails. Infections may become established in the palm, primarily, but infections here are more often secondary to spread of an infection from a finger tip, to the palm via the tendon sheath.

The edge of the finger nail is a common site for introduction of infection, as this area is often dirty and the site of small cuts or tears. Once infection is established here, it produces a characteristic abscess of the nail fold, known as a paronychia; this generally remains localised to the edge of the nail, occasionally spreading underneath the nail itself, and will usually respond to straightforward surgical treatment of the abscess, via incision and drainage under local anaesthesia.

On the palmar aspect of the finger tip, the pulp of the distal phalanx is another common area for infection and this produces a pulp abscess, or whitlow. These small abscesses are generally very painful, due to the tight nature of the tissues, and the patients generally seek advice very early, because of the tenderness and pain at the finger tip.

A long-standing infection at the finger tip, whether originating as a paronychia or pulp abscess, may eventually produce infection of the bone of the distal phalanx, although this usually only occurs in situations with a pre-disposing cause such as a retained foreign body, diabetic patient or other additional factor. Osteitis of the distal phalanx may be suspected from the long duration of the infection, the persistence of the infection despite apparently adequate incision and drainage, and the radiographic changes in the bone. If infection of the bone of the distal phalanx is suspected, the patient should be referred for further advice to an orthopaedic or hand surgery unit.

Most infections of the hand can be dealt with perfectly adequately in the accident and emergency department, but if the condition is not resolved within a few days a further opinion should be sought.

Infection in the Hand

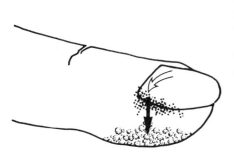

The most common site for localised infection in the hand is the side of the finger nail, a paronychia. Infection may spread from this site to the pulp of the finger, producing a pulp abscess or whitlow.

A pulp abscess, if untreated, may spread via the flexor tendon sheath to involve the palm of the hand and the deep spaces of the hand.

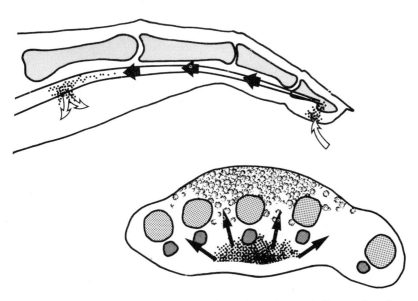

Because of the high pressure content of the palmar tissues, inflammation due to a palmar abscess generally presents as a swelling and redness on the dorsum of the hand, rather than in the palm itself.

TREATMENT OF THE INFECTED HAND

There is a widespread belief that treatment of infection in the hand consists of giving the patient antibiotics. While there are certainly situations where antibiotics are indicated, the majority of hand infections will resolve perfectly well, and indeed quicker, if treated with straightforward rest and elevation, followed by incision and drainage when appropriate. A patient presenting with an early infection in the hand, confined to the finger tip, is best treated by thorough splintage and elevation of the hand and this means not simply splinting the finger tip, but the entire finger and its neighbouring fingers, or if necessary the whole hand, and reviewing the patient again a day later. Most staphylococcal infections will either settle spontaneously or proceed to abscess formation with this type of splintage and elevation, and once pus has formed, then incision of the abscess will relieve the pain and allow the abscess to heal spontaneously. Antibiotic therapy for this straightforward type of infection offers no advantages, and the only indication for it in this situation is when the infection is spreading. If the patient is complaining of pain severe enough to keep him awake at night, then this generally means that there is pus present in the infection and indeed the pus itself may be visible or the abscess may be palpable as a fluctuant centre of an inflammatory area. Surgical drainage should be carried out under adequate anaesthesia, and a proximal local anaesthetic block is ideal for most hand infections, although for a large infection in the palm of the hand, a general anaesthetic may be preferable. There is a traditional belief that local anaesthetic should not be used in the presence of infection, but this relates to the use of local infiltration anaesthesia and certainly injecting lignocaine in the local region of an abscess would be most unwise, as it would encourage the spread of the infection, but properly carried out nerve block in normal tissues, proximal to the infection, will give rise to no complications. The use of a tourniquet is not necessary when draining an abscess, and indeed is contra-indicated, as an attempt at exsanguinating a limb may spread the infection.

There are a large number of important structures in the hand which lie superficially, such as tendons and digital nerves, and an incision in the hand must be carefully judged so as to avoid damaging these structures. In general, a longitudinal incision in the finger or hand, over the point of maximal fluctuation of the abscess will avoid any significant structures, although such an incision should not be taken across a joint flexion crease. If the abscess formation involves bone, tendon sheath, or any of the deep palmar spaces in the hand, then further advice should be sought, as incision of this more serious infection should not be attempted in the accident and emergency department. Excision of an abscess in the hand should be via a generous incision, and if necrotic skin lies over the abscess this should be excised, leaving a saucer shaped hole to allow full clearance of the underlying pus.

Treatment of the Infected Hand

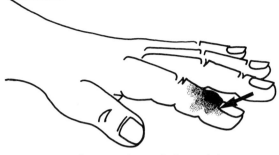

Once an abscess is formed the treatment is surgical. The abscess should be drained through an adequate incision and all pus allowed to drain. The common paronychia should be drained by a longitudinal incision along the edge of the nail bed.

In the early stages of infection, and also following incision and drainage, the finger, and indeed the whole hand, should be comfortably splinted and elevated, as this will reduce the pain and swelling of the infection.

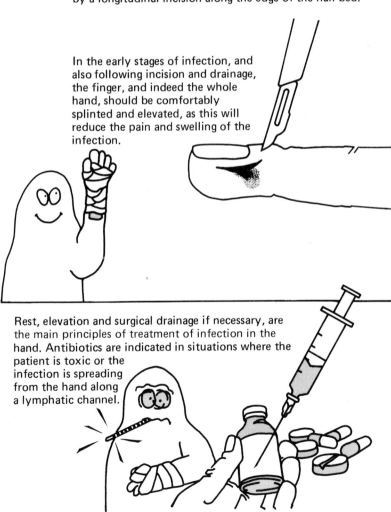

Rest, elevation and surgical drainage if necessary, are the main principles of treatment of infection in the hand. Antibiotics are indicated in situations where the patient is toxic or the infection is spreading from the hand along a lymphatic channel.

In a small minority of cases, the infecting organisms will be other than staphylococcal:

1. Where the infection is obviously spreading up the forearm, and particularly where there is evidence of lymphangitis, a red line running up the forearm to the elbow and up to the axilla, this strongly suggests the presence of streptococcal infection which is very much more prone to spread and is less liable to cause abscess formation. Streptococcal organisms have remained sensitive to penicillin and if this type of infection is suspected, then treatment with straightforward crystalline penicillin, or its oral equivalent, should be perfectly effective.

2. Where there has been a suggestion of human or animal tooth bites causing the initiating wound, it is likely that the bacterial flora will be very mixed, and will include a number of unusual organisms such as *Pasteurella septica*, *Actinomyces* and *Bacteroides*. In this situation a broad spectrum antibiotic is recommended, together with thorough debridement or excision of the original wound to remove the source of these organisms.

3. Burns of the hand, like burns elsewhere on the body, are particularly prone to infection with some gram negative organisms such as *Proteus* and *Pyocyaneus*. If this type of infection does occur, then the patient should be referred to a specialised burns centre, as eradication of this infection requires careful and intensive treatment, and the infection itself will prevent the burn from healing.

4. Some occupational diseases may present as infections in the hand, for example orf is a viral disease associated with sheep and sheep farming, and patients in this sort of occupation may present with areas of small clear lesions in the hand, which, when they burst, may become secondarily infected, usually with staphylocci. Anthrax, although rare, may occur as a classical malignant pustule on the hands of patients working with hides or similar animal products imported from abroad.

PERSISTENT INFECTION

Most hand infections will clear up promptly and easily under good treatment, but if patients return with repeated infection, or the initial infection refuses to subside properly, then other causes should be looked for. Repeated infection may be self-inflicted, for example in drug addicts who are in the habit of breaking the skin with needle punctures, often in less than ideal conditions. Patients on steroid therapy, and diabetics, often unaware of the diabetes, will be liable to repeated infection or difficulty in clearing an apparently straightforward infection. A malignant melanoma underneath the finger nail, the sub-ungual variety, may appear very much like a paronychia initially, and if a simple infection of the finger nail fails to respond to straightforward surgical drainage, the possibility of such an underlying tumour should be borne in mind.

A further cause for a persisting infection despite apparently adequate treatment, is the presence of a foreign body in the wound, and a careful history of the initial injury, together with appropriate X-ray examination, should be sufficient to establish whether any foreign material still remains in the wound.

TETANUS

Tetanus infections should not be a problem in populations where active immunisation is available to children. It is standard practice in British hospitals to consider all open wounds to be at risk from tetanus organisms, and to cover patients with a single dose of tetanus toxoid and a long-acting penicillin, unless a confident history of immune status exists. In countries or populations where tetanus immunisation is not standard, it would be prudent to carry out a more extensive debridement and cleaning of wounds, especially agricultural ones, than is advocated in this book. The patient should be encouraged to acquire tetanus immunity via a course of toxoid injections, but with a significantly contaminated wound, a brief course of passive immunisation, using human anti-toxin, may be advisable.

Chapter 9

BURNS

The majority of burns of the hand seen in an accident department are straightforward thermal or electrical burns. There are, however, some unusual types of burn which are described at the end of this section.

Thermal burns, whether due to flame burns or scalds, tend to produce a broad area of relatively superficial damage—the essential point to decide is whether there has been any significant area of whole thickness necrosis of the skin. If the full thickness of the skin has not been damaged, then the burn will heal, in time, leaving little or no scar or other damage. Such superficial burns generally produce an area of painful and tender erythema and blistering. The treatment of superficial partial thickness burns consists essentially of dressing the burn to minimise infection, and splinting the hand to prevent awkward contractures. Most burns will exude serum for a day or two, and excising the blisters is easily done and makes subsequent dressings simpler; a tulle gras (Xeroform, Jelonet) dressing impregnated with chlorhexidine or a broad spectrum antibiotic is advisable to minimise secondary infection, and the hand and fingers should be splinted comfortably in the position of function, and elevated for the first day or two.

All burns produce oedema and swelling, and in the hand this tends to lead to stiffness and slow return of function; it is therefore important to splint the hand comfortably in a good position during the initial stages of the treatment (see page 68).

The severity of a burn is proportional to the size of the damaged and necrotic area; in a flame burn or scald the surface area of skin damage is important, and with an electrical burn, the depth of the burn is more important and difficult to determine.

If the full thickness of the skin has been burned, then the skin cannot regenerate and healing by scar will eventually occur. This scar is unsightly, but of more significance as far as the use of the hand is concerned, is that this scar generally produces troublesome contractures of fingers and joints. Any full thickness burn greater than 2 cm in size should therefore be referred for further advice from a hand or plastic surgeon. An area of full thickness burn may be recognised as a pale and insensitive area of skin, usually surrounded by a red, inflamed and tender area of partial thickness burn.

Electrical burns of the hand can be misleading—they appear to be small in size, but they are generally very deep, with damage to all layers down to and including bone and joint.

Chemical burns are generally treated in industrial medical centres, which are aware of specific antidotes to locally used chemicals; in general, chemical burns should be washed with a copious amount of water until knowledge of the specific chemical and its treatment is available. Hydrofluoric acid, used in the glass

98

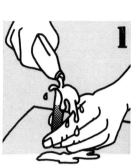
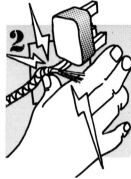
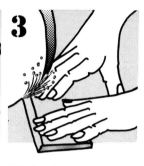

Chemical burn: use specific antidote initially and then treat as flame burn.

Electric burn: small in area but very deep. There is often much more damage than one initially suspects.

Friction burns: generally very dirty wounds, but the damage is all visible.

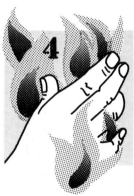
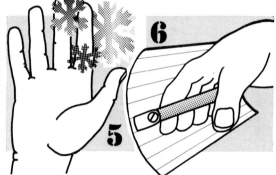

Flame burns, or scalds: relatively large area of superficial damage. Dressings to partial thickness burns, excision and grafting of full thickness burns.

Frostbite: adopt a conservative policy, as these often heal remarkably well.

Radiator burns: especially in children, produce awkward full thickness burns on the volar aspect of the fingers leading to difficult contractures.

and etching trades, can cause extremely painful burns of the hand, and this pain can be neutralised by small subcutaneous injections of calcium gluconate into the burned area, as the calcium ion fixes the damaging hydrogen fluoride.

Radiation burns are unusual, and any suggestion of damage caused by a radioactive source must be referred immediately to the local radiation protection officer.

Frostbite, due to extremes of low temperature and exposure, can cause necrosis of extremities, feet, hands and ears particularly. Local treatment is of little avail, and the patient with frostbite should be admitted to hospital for general resuscitation and assessment. Frostbitten fingers generally take some weeks to demarcate the damaged area, but in the end often heal remarkably well.

Chapter 10

MEDICO-LEGAL PROBLEMS

Working at the front door of a hospital, in the accident unit, is a particularly responsible situation, and the possibility of a missed diagnosis or inappropriate treatment must always be at the back of one's mind. In this book we have tried to point out some of the more obvious or serious pitfalls when dealing with the injured hand. The most certain way of avoiding trouble is to listen to the patient, examine him properly, and make careful notes. Such clinical notes need not necessarily be extensive, but you should certainly make a note of what the patient tells you was the cause of the accident, what his complaint is, and the basic elements of your findings on examination. If the patient has any type of laceration or cut on the hand, you *must* make a comment on function of tendons and nerves.

If there is any possibility of a fracture or joint injury, or of a foreign body in the hand, it must be X-rayed. Patients, and lawyers, put a lot of weight on the taking of an X-ray, even if it is completely negative, and it is best to have a negative radiograph and a satisfied patient rather than no radiograph and a patient who is still worrying that his hand may be broken.

Throughout this book we have stressed the use of the telephone to ask advice from senior colleagues; diagnosis of injuries in the hand is generally simple and straightforward, certainly to someone with some experience in the field, and if you lack the experience, then you should be asking for help.

The patient who attends an accident unit with an injured hand should leave the department satisfied and comfortable; if it is a simple problem then the diagnosis should be clear and the treatment straightforward; a more significant injury may have been treated in the accident unit, in which case the patient should be looking forward to returning to his occupation within 3 weeks or so, while, if it is likely to take longer than this, or if the diagnosis is unclear, then advice should have been sought from a senior colleague or a referral for such an opinion organised.

DATE	
	NAME	HOSPITAL No.	
		AGE	
	PHYS.	DEPT.	
	SURG.	WARD	

HAND SURGERY

DIAGNOSIS:

AETIOLOGY:

ANAESTHETIC:

OPERATIVE FINDINGS:— SKIN? TENDON? NERVE? JOINT?

REPAIR PROCEDURE:

SURGEON:

SPLINTAGE: FOLLOW UP:

JMcC/9776

This type of hand examination record will minimise the risk of a missed diagnosis.

Chapter 11

COMMON PITFALLS

CASE 1

Question:
Have you any comments to make on this case record?

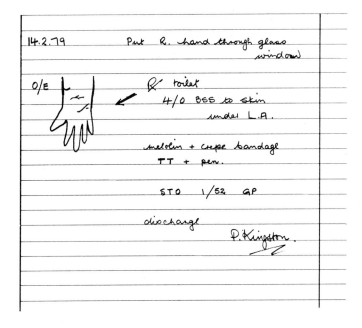

14.2.79   Put R. hand through glass
                                    window

O/E   ✗ toilet
              4/0 BSS to skin
                  under L.A.

            melolin + crepe bandage
            TT + pen.

            STO   1/52   GP

            discharge
                        P. Kingston.

CASE 1

Answer:

Anyone who puts their hand through a glass window has almost certainly cut a number of tendons and nerves.

There is no comment in this case record of any clinical examination of tendons or nerves in the hand.

Suturing skin with silk sutures produces a fair result, but the use of 4/0, 5/0 or 6/0 (1.5, 1, 0.7 metric) monofilament nylon or prolene is preferable.

Melolin (Telfa) is an inappropriate type of dressing for the hand.

With the number of lacerations shown on this hand, it would have been better splinted for the first few postoperative days.

This patient returned 2 weeks later to the hand clinic with a quite obvious complete division of his median nerve, and partial division of two flexor tendons to the fingers. This is just the type of patient who should be carefully examined in the accident unit, and if any suspicion of damage to tendons or nerves is found should be referred for proper primary care by a skilled hand surgeon.

CASE 2

Question:

This patient received a burn of her hand when a faulty bedside light exploded in her hand. What do you think might be damaged in this hand, and how might it be treated?

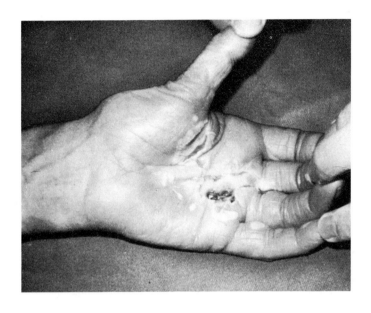

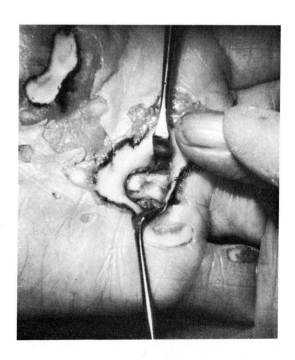

Answer:

The upper photograph shows the necrotic tendons, both super-ficial and profundus, which were removed from the palm of the hand, and there was similar damage to the digital nerves to the ring finger. In this situation, attempted repair or reconstruction of tendons and nerves to a ring finger is inadvisable, and a straight-forward primary amputation of the ring finger was carried out and the wound healed in 2 weeks' time. Note that the burn at the base of the thenar eminence, which had not affected any tendons or nerves, was treated by excision of the damaged skin and primary skin graft.

The lower photograph on the previous page shows well the appearance of full thickness skin loss with a surrounding area of partial thickness loss, characteristic of an electric burn.

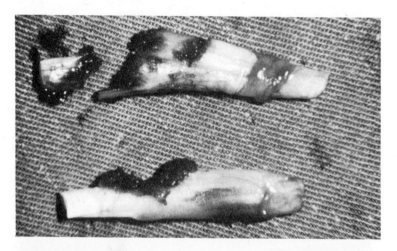

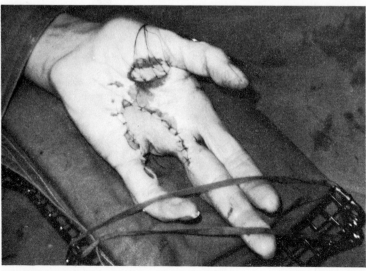

CASE 3

Question:
This boy fell while delivering milk and cut his hand on a milk bottle. What do you suspect may be damaged in the hand?

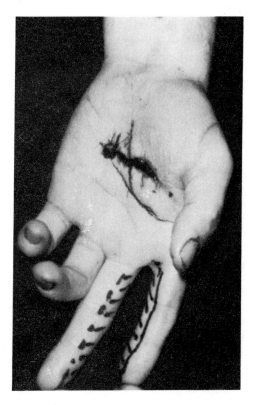

CASE 3

Answer:

The careful examining doctor has appreciated that there was loss of sensation on the sides of the index/middle finger cleft, and at surgical exploration the severed ends of the digital nerves to these two fingers were found. Primary repair of these digital nerves by means of a few fine 8/0 (0.4 metric) nylon sutures was carried out on the day of injury and good recovery of sensation occurred over the following months. Despite the extended attitude of the index and middle fingers on the previous photograph, the flexor tendons to these fingers were clinically intact.

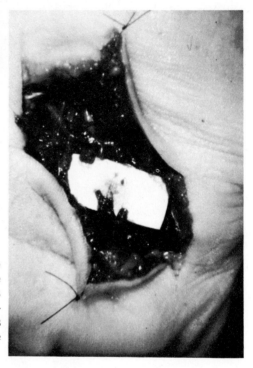

CASE 4

Question:
This 11-year-old girl suffered superficial flame burns to the chest and right forearm and hand two days prior to the photograph. Have you any comments to make on the treatment to date or in the future?

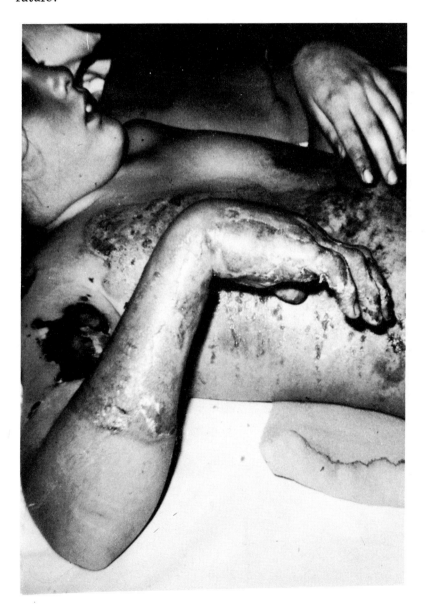

CASE 4

Answer:

The burned right hand is a classic example of poor splintage. The hand has been allowed to fall into flexion at the wrist, and the metacarpophalangeal joints are extended, and the fingers, if left in this position, will develop very intractable clawing. Since the burns were essentially partial thickness, confident healing of the skin could be expected, and treatment was concentrated on the position of the hand. The two photographs on this page illustrate the splintage used in this particular case to obtain the position of function in the hand, and the results two weeks after the initial photograph with the skin steadily healing and the hand in a good position. The eventual function in this hand was normal.

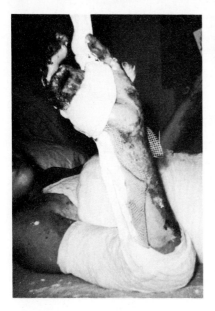
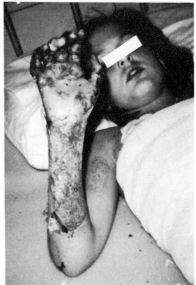

CASE 5

Question:

This woman fell on a broken glass at a party. What structures are likely to have been damaged in her hand?

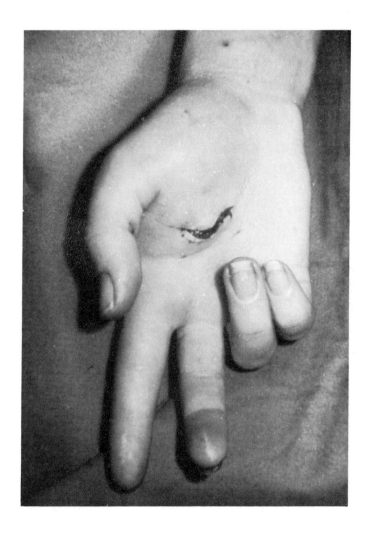

CASE 5

Answer:

Do not assume that the broken glass went into the hand in a straightforward vertical fashion; it may have entered in any direction, and certainly from first examination of the hand it should be obvious that both flexor tendons to the index finger have been cut and probably the superficial tendon to the middle finger. Other structures which should be tested for:

(1) Digital nerves to the radial side of the index finger, the index finger/middle finger cleft, and the middle finger/ring finger cleft.
(2) The motor branch of the median nerve.
(3) Digital nerves to both sides of the thumb.
(4) The flexor pollicis longus tendon.
(5) The deep motor branch of the ulnar nerve as it runs across the palm.

It may not be possible to ascertain the continuity of all of these structures but this hand should be submitted to careful, formal exploration in an operating theatre by a competent hand surgeon.

CASE 6

Question:
The ring on this lady's finger caught in a moving door with this
result. What would be your management?

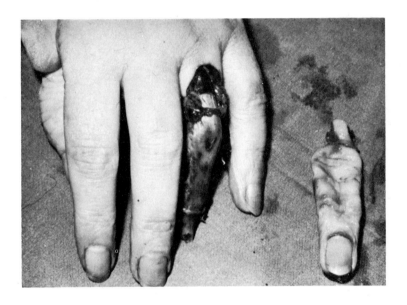

CASE 6

Answer:

This finger should be amputated, probably via a metacarpo-phalangeal disarticulation. Replacement of the de-gloved skin as a free graft would certainly fail, and even microsurgery would be of no avail here because of the marked damage to fine vessels, which can be seen as a mottling of the skin of the finger, and is generally of bad prognostic significance when considering replantation.

Theoretically one can clothe the stripped finger with skin, via complex pedicle flaps, but the resultant function and appearance of the finger would be very poor indeed, and in this case amput-ation was carried out, the stump healing within a week or two, and the resultant function of the hand as a whole is excellent, the patient is well-satisfied.

CASE 7

Question:
This patient attended the dressing clinic with a wound on the back of his hand which is healing well. Have you any comments to make?

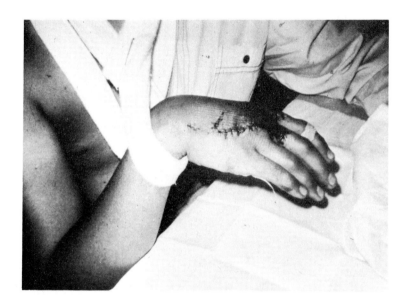

CASE 7

Answer:

This is another example of bad or inappropriate splinting of the hand. This type of 'Collar and Cuff' splintage is never suitable for hand injuries. It positively encourages the wrist to flex and the fingers to extend at the metacarpophalangeal joints, and in a position such as this, even a hand with a minor injury is liable to develop troublesome stiffness. If you intend to splint the hand it is best to splint the forearm, wrist, hand and a number of fingers in the position of function, and if you wish to elevate the hand it is better to use a triangular bandage, or broad arm sling, rather than this type of support.

CASE 8

Question:

Following a laceration at the base of the right index and middle fingers, this seaman attended a hand surgery unit complaining of loss of movement and sensation in the two fingers. This photograph shows the relevant anatomy at exploratory surgery—can you identify any structures here?

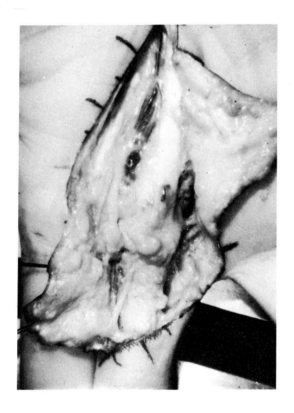

CASE 8

Answer:

Apparently some divided structures had been noted in the accident unit which he first attended, and he was told the tendons had been repaired. This photograph shows the sort of problems caused by inexperienced attempts at repairing tendons or nerves. The flexor tendons to the middle finger are completely bound down by dense scar tissue, and the suture material, which appeared to be 3/0 (2.0 metric) silk, was extruding from the tendon and was totally inappropriate for this type of repair. Furthermore, the digital nerves which had been divided had obviously not been recognised, and at least two of them had been sutured into the tendon anastomosis.

If you suspect damage to flexor tendons or digital nerves in the hand or fingers, and the facilities or surgeons to repair these structures are not available, then it is far better to simply suture the skin, splint the hand, and refer the patient to the nearest competent unit. Disentangling this sort of mess makes life difficult for everyone and makes a satisfactory end result extremely unlikely.

CASE 9

Question:
These two photographs show the clinical and radiological appearance of a thumb after a fall while ski-ing. Any comments?

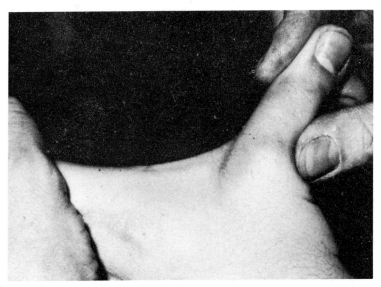

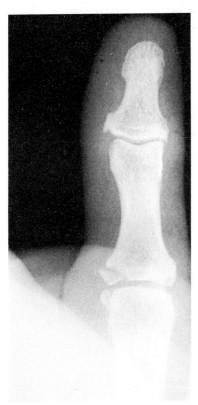

CASE 9

Answer:

A classical example of rupture of the ulnar collateral ligament of the metacarpophalangeal joint of the thumb due to forced abduction of the thumb. This commonly occurs in ski-ing and other similar sports where a fall on the outstretched thumb may occur. If the fragment is small and the instability not severe, conservative treatment in a plaster cast will suffice, but in this case the collateral ligament had pulled off a significant fracture of bone, shown in the upper photograph, and formal surgical repair of this damaged ligament was carried out with an excellent result 3 months later. Failure to recognise or treat this type of injury leads to chronic weakness and instability of the thumb, and a weak power grip in the hand.

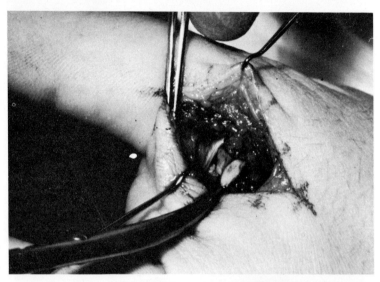

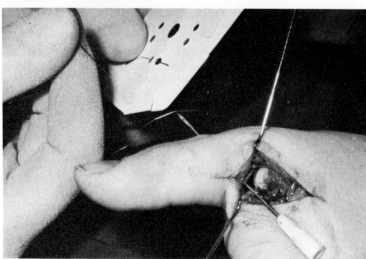

CASE 10

Question:
How would you describe this radiograph and how would you consider treating the injury?

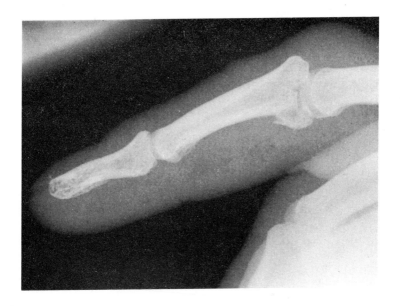

CASE 10

Answer:

This is an articular fracture of the proximal interphalangeal joint, with a detached volar fragment at the base of the middle phalanx. It is important to appreciate that there has been significant dorsal subluxation of the middle phalanx on the head of the proximal phalanx. One can also appreciate considerable soft tissue swelling around the joint due to a haematoma formation.

It is not possible to reduce and hold this fracture dislocation in a reduced position by a closed method, and either pinning the joint with a Kirschner wire, or formal open exploration of the joint and careful reconstruction of the bones using small fragment fixation, will be necessary in order to achieve a useful range of movement in this joint.

CASE 11

Question:
Fracture occurred during a game of football and has been treated by immobilisation of the finger in a malleable aluminium splint. Have you any comment to make?

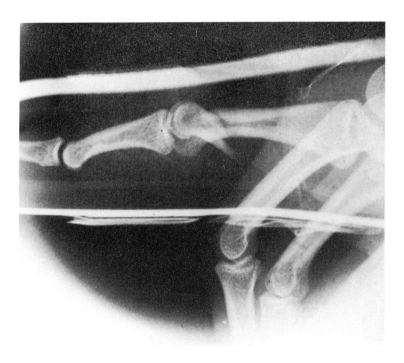

Answer:

There are hardly any indications for splinting a finger fully extended, and splinting a single finger, with this kind of aluminium splintage, is generally worse than useless. This fracture involves two-thirds of the head of the proximal phalanx, and it must be appreciated that the function of the proximal interphalangeal joint is very much at risk. The spike of bone is also likely to be interfering with the function of the long flexor tendon.

The photograph on this page shows the final result in this case, with a grossly deranged proximal interphalangeal joint which had virtually no movement in it, and the flexor tendon was also completely stuck to the bone of the proximal phalanx and altogether this finger was almost useless due to poor initial diagnosis and treatment.

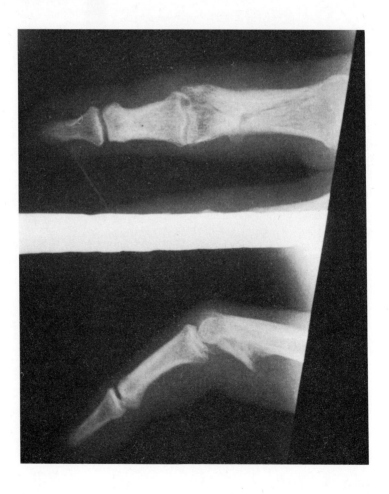

CASE 12

Question:

This motor mechanic was lubricating a vehicle when he hurt his left little finger. It had become increasingly painful over a period of 2 hours and he presented in the accident unit.

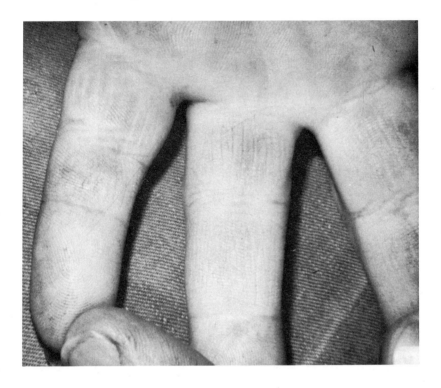

CASE 12

Answer:

Exploration of the base of the little finger revealed a considerable quantity of black grease lying in the subcutaneous tissues and around the flexor tendon to the little finger. Prompt removal of this material, followed by splintage of the hand and supervised mobilisation resulted in normal function of this finger.

Refer back to the previous photograph and appreciate the virtually insignificant entry wound which can just be seen in the ring/little finger cleft.

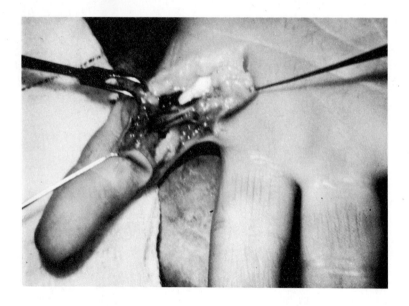

Here is another photograph of a high pressure injection entry wound, in a left index finger tip, in this case due to the protective wax which is sprayed over cars before delivery. This wax had penetrated the flexor tendon sheath and complete exposure of the entire tendon and tendon sheath was necessary together with washing out of the tendon sheath, in order to remove as much of the foreign material as possible. Despite this prompt action, this patient ended up with a somewhat stiff index finger, although he was able to return to work eventually.

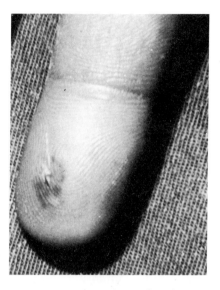

Any delay in dealing with these injuries, even for a few hours, allows the toxic materials to become fixed to the tissues and loss of a finger or part of the hand may result.

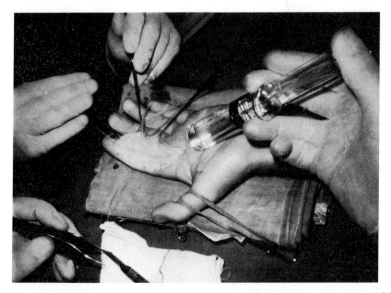

FURTHER READING

This book is purely an introduction to traumatic hand surgery, and a guide to diagnosis and treatment in the accident unit. There are a number of other books which deal with various aspects of the injured hand in more detail, and some suggestions for further reading are:

An Illustrated Handbook in Local Anaesthesia Ed. Eriksson; Munksgaard, Copenhagen, Denmark, 1969.

This is a beautifully illustrated and very lucid instructional book on all varieties and techniques of local anaesthesia.

The Care of Minor Hand Injuries A. Flatt; C.V. Mosby, St Louis, Missouri, USA, 1972.

Treatment of Hand Injuries E. Weckesser; Year Book Medical Publishers, Chicago, USA, 1974.

These two books cover the same general topics as this small volume, but in much greater detail. They are designed for the accident surgeon who wishes to deal with certain bone and tendon injuries, for example, and has the facilities available for this type of surgery. As in this book, these authors advise caution in trying to achieve too much in the emergency room/accident unit.

The Hand: Diagnosis & Indications G. Lister; Churchill Livingstone, Edinburgh, Scotland, 1978.

For the doctor uncertain how to examine tendons and nerves, this book is a mine of information; all aspects of examination of the hand, and not only the injured hand, are well described and illustrated.

Fundamental Techniques of Plastic Surgery I. McGregor; Churchill Livingstone, Edinburgh, Scotland, 1972.

Respect for, and care of, the tissues of the hand, including suturing and grafting techniques are clearly described in this book.

Fractures Vol. 1. C.A. Rockwood and D.P. Green; J.B. Lippincott, Philadelphia, USA, 1972.

The chapter on fractures and dislocations in the hand is an excellent review of the subject, with sound conclusions and suggestions for treating both simple and difficult injuries.